Short St Meta

by John Smale

Metaphors and stories for changing the way we understand life, the World and our feelings.

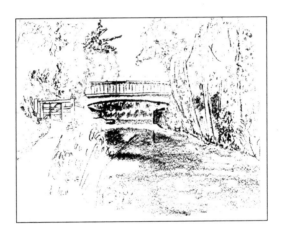

Metaphors are tools for change.
They break the barriers of rigid thinking.
They empower us to think in a lateral way.
They illuminate the way forward to a better path.
They help us to recognise the causes of our problems.
Metaphors enable us to create new patterns of thought.

This book is a work of fiction. The names, characters and incidents in this book are the work of the author's imagination. Any resemblance to any persons living or dead or any locations or scenarios are purely coincidental.

Published in September 2008 by emp3books, Kiln Workshops, Pilcot Road, Crookham Village, Fleet, Hampshire, GU51 5RY, England

Previously published by Exposure Publishing 2007

ISBN-10: 0-9550736-3-4
ISBN-13: 978-0-9550736-3-2

www.emp3books.com

CONTENTS

The stories have themes, which address modern views of ourselves and others. The intention is to encourage personal insights into our own problems and attitudes in order to encourage positive personal changes.

ANIMAL NATURE
We can see reflections of ourselves in the characters of animals. The wolf in 'Little Red Riding Hood' represents the predatory nature of men. The dragons that needed to be slayed were, and are, the threats from bullies. Sometimes people, sometimes nations.

The stories that follow in this section include animals to symbolise the pressures of life. Our need to strive to advance at the expense of happiness. Our erroneous beliefs about others, including nature.

6.   The Salmon's Story. The choice between risk and safety in our search for fulfilment.

7.   The Frog's Ladder. Whilst helping others is good, making total sacrifices is counter productive.

8.   The Hawk's Story. Sometimes the discovery of liberation is frightening. The freedom that is gained should be welcomed rather than feared.

9.   The Fly's Story. Is about not understanding what is really good for us.

10.   The Web. Shows that creativity and individuality, as well as logic, have a place in the advancement of our lives.

HUMAN NATURE

Anger, revenge, prejudice and dominance seem to be primeval drives. However, they pervade modern life. These are human failings over which we have control, if we think about the consequences for ourselves, and others.

11. Rejection. Describes a need by some people who feel that they have been rejected, to reject others. By doing so, they feel that they have eliminated the possibility that they will be rejected again.

12. Poisoning The Well. Deliberate revenge often returns to hurt the revenger.

13. The Precious Vase. Tells us that we do have choices when it comes to the actions taken whilst angry.

14. The Fisherman's Story. There is a need to let go of what is broken before we become damaged ourselves.

15. Surfing Life. How to take control of our own destinies in a world that seems determined to govem our lives for us.

16. Who Or What. Is about the faulty nature of prejudice. We should reserve opinions until we understand who the person is rather than assume from the first impression.

17. The Third Eye. Is about the cruelty of mankind to itself, other creatures and the world.

18. Magic. Is about how selfishness works against the individual rather than for him. It explains how the desire to help only ourselves leads to finding nothing but disappointment.

19. The Scapegoat's Story. Highlights the pointless need to assign blame to others.

NATURE'S NATURE

Nature is not something that exists outside our windows. We live in nature. We exist on a living planet that we have a greater need for than it has for us. We should treat the world as if were really our mother rather than something than needs to be destroyed for profits.

20. The Mood Rainbow. We can look at things in two ways, the positive and the negative. The colours of the rainbow come from pure light. When those colours are mixed they make a gloomy mess.

21. The Wind-Blasted Tree. Explains how we can form negative attitudes towards ourselves that are different to the reality of how we are perceived by others.

22. The Volcano's Story. Tells of the destructive effects of uncontrolled violence.

23. The River's Story. Is about remorse.

24. Straight Lines. Continues the theme that logic has been sold as the correct way to think, whereas nature has no rules of precision in its beauty.

25. The Water-Wheel. Looks at the innocent recycling that occurs in a simple way.

26. The Wave's Story. The cycle of energy told as a story about a wave in the ocean.

INSIGHT TO ANGER

A continuing narrative about anger the causes, effects and resolution of anger.

27. The Angry Man

28. Blame

29. Killing The Anger

30. Power

31. Judgement

32. The New Domain

33. Time

34. The Four Parts

35. Resolution

INTRODUCTION

We live in a stressful world. Very often we live at a distance from the people who we could ask for help or advice. Regrettably, it is often easier to recognise the causes and effects of problems after the event, with the benefit of hindsight. Therefore, these short stories, based on real-life experiences, have been written in order to offer help to people who are suffering, or who might suffer, from negative influences in their lives.

The stories are based on the adverse effects that behaviours, attitudes and actions have had on the lives of others. Therefore, if the listeners can benefit from recognising symptoms of their own issues that have caused problems, then there is the possibility that they can take corrective action before suffering strikes them.

Of course, it would be wonderful if we all had access to a wise sage who could point us in the right direction from time to time.

With these stories you can imagine that you have travelled back in time to the site of a storyteller's circle. During our early years we gained our view of the world which contains us by listening to our parents, grandparents, teachers and even by watching children's television. The world we built then is still within us.

The art of a storyteller is to use that world to create analogies, examples and metaphors in a world in which animals and plants appear to think and act as humans. In this way we can learn afresh by looking at ourselves from a new perspective.

ANIMAL NATURE

1. THE OLD STORY TELLER

In very old times there was a revered storyteller who travelled from village to village to share his understanding of life. He had seen and experienced so many happy and sad things in his, and others' lives. Because he was a kind and caring person he wanted others to share the delights that life can offer by avoiding the sorrow that can very often occur instead.

He had learnt that quoting real events was like offering advice that had little effect at all because there was no participation in the incident by the listener. So, instead he told his stories as metaphors and similes that had to be interpreted by the audience. As he said once, "I will give you a present, but you have to unwrap it in order to see its value."

Those tales have been preserved and are now re-told. It is likely that he would have enjoyed knowing that his good intentions have been given extra life. Read them, uncover their meanings, and adapt them to your own life. The aim is to bring you clear reasons for positive changes, but you must allow yourself time to ponder upon the information that they contain.

Imagine that you have moved way back in time where you are sitting in a small circle of people, around a big fire in the twilight of a lovely sunny day. You are in-between the face of a hill that has the entrances to a number of caves, and the start of a pine forest.

The sparks from the fire floating into the dusky sky seem to blend with the bright stars shining from the heavens above. Your breathing is slow and deep, and you close your eyes in order to concentrate upon the sounds around you. Imagine that you can hear the crackling of the fire, and the rustling of some birds settling down for the evening while others are preparing for the night.

The air is warm and scented by the pine in the woods. You are seated on the sandy ground that feels soft and slightly dusty when you run your fingers over it.

A ragged old man with white hair and a long matted white beard moves into the circle. He looks around with his sharp eyes peering through weather-aged eyelids. His leathery skin is tanned and his sacking tunic torn. He looks so worn and tired but his presence is bewildering.

Allow yourself to enjoy his stories through your imagination, allow yourself to be transported to the scene of every story.

2. THE BIRD'S WORLDS

The world seemed a hard place. The world seemed to be a cramped place. The world was certainly dark place.

But the world was a warm and safe place. Despite everything that we can think, it was the only world that the bird knew. Day after day there was nothing to do except relax and grow. There was no need to search for food because it was there. There was no need to do anything because everything happened automatically.

But this world was also a boring place. There was not much to do, nothing to see. However, it was warm and safe.

The bird wanted something to happen. It wanted adventure. It wanted its world to be bigger. It felt the time was right to start exploring.

It tapped the edge of its world with its beak. Then it tapped again. Suddenly there was a sharp, cracking noise. The bird had broken the world. It was shocked. Then a piece fell away and there were more splintering noises and a bright light broke the darkness.

The destruction of the world gave the bird more room. It could move its legs and stumpy wings. As it did so, more of the boundary fell away. The chick was perplexed. It felt guilty that it had broken its orb. It felt worried about the afterlife. For the first time ever, it felt vulnerable.

The chick struggled to pick up the pieces of shell to rebuild the egg, but they were being discarded by a huge monster with a large beak and staring eyes.

Suddenly it was free from the world that it knew. It had moved on.

This world seemed a soft place. This world seemed to be an open place. This world was certainly a light place.

But this world was a warm and safe place. Despite everything that we can think, it was the only world that the bird knew, now. Day after day there was nothing to do except relax, grow and play-fight with its brothers and sisters. There was no need to search for food because it was there. There was no need to do anything because everything happened automatically. Every-so-often a huge spike would ram food down its gaping beak.

But this world was also a boring place. There was not much to do apart from exercising its wings. There was nothing to see apart from the leaves that surrounded the nest. However, it was warm and safe.

The bird wanted something to happen. It wanted adventure. It wanted its world to be bigger. It felt the time was right to start exploring. It wondered if there was something outside this new shell.

One day it climbed onto the edge of the nest and flapped its wings. The next day it did the same, but it fell. As it heard the cracking of twigs, it thought that it had smashed this new world. As it plummeted, its wings suddenly slowed its descent. Then when it flapped them it started to move upwards.

Suddenly it was free from the world that it knew. It had moved on.

The destruction of the second world gave the bird more room. It could move its legs and wings. The young bird was perplexed. It felt guilty that it had broken this new world. It felt worried about the afterlife. For the second time in its life, it felt vulnerable. It glided to the ground and looked around.

A snake lunged at the bird and swallowed it.

This third world seemed a hard place. This world seemed to be a cramped place. This world was certainly dark place. But this world seemed to be a warm and safe place. But this world was also a boring place. There was not much to do, nothing to see.

The bird wanted something to happen. It wanted adventure. It wanted its world to be bigger. It felt the time was right to start exploring but it could not move. The bird wished that it had stayed in the egg. The bird wished that it had stayed in the nest.

As it died, it wondered what the next world would be like after it had smashed this one.

3. THE SNAKE'S SKIN

The snake slithered through the undergrowth. It was beautiful. The patches of sunlight highlighted the colours of its scales. Reds, blues and greens of different shades seemed to shine like jewels. The snake was so proud of its skin. Other snakes were envious. Those that were dull to look at were often sarcastic because they felt less impressive. The snake took their comments to be praise. Its skin was thick as well as imposing.

However, as the snake grew, its skin became tighter and tighter. It was uncomfortable but the snake was determined to retain its advantage. The stretching made the skin less attractive, but it was still better than the others.

The tautness made it difficult for the snake to catch its prey so it did not grow as quickly as it should have done, so in a very strange way, the snake was able to retain its good looks for longer, so it was happy.

One day, as the snake was attempting to cross an open space, a huge eagle swooped down, picked it up in its talons and flew to a tree to eat its meal. The snake, so upset with this effrontery, hissed so loudly that the eagle loosened its grip. The snake wriggled and fell to the ground. It found a small hole to hide in.

Later, when it felt safer, it emerged. Inspecting its skin, it noticed little rips and tears. Its skin was splitting open.

Devastated that its pride and joy was about to be lost, the snake sneaked out of sight. As it did, its loose skin caught on a thorn. As the snake tried to free itself, the remainder of its old skin was pulled off.

The snake hid away for many days until hunger drove it to go hunting. It was seen by another snake that hissed and gasped. It said, "There used to be a snake around here that had the most beautiful skin. We haven't seen it for a while after it was caught by an eagle. But, if it were still around, it would be so jealous of you. That is the most wonderful snake-skin I have ever seen."

The snake was shocked. It had been too worried to look at its new skin, too ashamed to have lost so much splendour.

It reared up and looked at itself. Having not seen so much glory before, it was shocked at the improvement. It wondered why it had tried so hard to retain something that was obscuring something that was so much better.

Now it knew that the process of life involved losing things that we have outgrown, knowing that the future will always be better than the past.

4. THE FISH POND

The fish pond was quite big. It was big enough to allow a large amount of diversity in plant and aquatic life.

The fish saw their world for what it was. The sky was the surface of the water. The bottom of the pond was the limit of their planet. Beyond the sky there were other planets from which aliens would appear. Some were friendly, especially the green aliens that would lay their eggs in huge bundles. These eggs would be offered as food gifts to the fish. Then some would turn into black wriggly things that swam like fish, but were different. These were good to eat as well.

However, some of the aliens were hostile. The huge grey ones would stand on the sky and would spear the fish from time to time. That was horrible, and caused quite a lot of panic.

The baby fish were attacked by black monsters in suits of armour, sometimes.

But there seemed to be a God. Now and again the fish would seem to see his face smiling from above the sky. He dropped food onto the sky that they would swim up to eat. The religious fish called this "Matter from Heaven."

The fish wondered what life was like outside their world. They tried to talk to the frogs, but they could not establish a language for communication. The frogs would either be mating or hiding. They didn't really seem to belong there.

And, the Great Diving Beetles were too repulsive to want to get to know.

There were newts from time to time that would arrive to gobble up all sorts of food from the fish eggs to bits of mud, or so it seemed. They were no great company, either.

A lot of time was spent in intellectual debate on the meaning of life and whether God really did exist or not. Even though he appeared on a regular basis, he did not seem to do much to give a quality of life to the fish, apart from dropping the bits of food that supplemented their diet.

Sometimes, when one of the fish became ill, it would be taken up by the Net-of-God. Perhaps it might return, but usually it did not.

A lot of time was spent discussing what happened to the fish that were taken by God.

Were they put into a huge pond free from aliens, where food would be abundant and the water fresh and well oxygenated?

Or were they tortured and kept in a small plastic bag like the ones that were seen sometimes when new fish arrived? There was no way to know.

It was assumed, however, that the fish that had been good were more likely to be placed into the blissful world, and those that had been bad…well.

But God seemed to be too remote. He only seemed to answer prayers, sometimes. For example, when the pond became hot in the summer and more oxygen was needed, the fish would go to the sky, look upwards to where God appeared to appear sometimes and they would mouth prayers for air.

This didn't work every time. Some days the 'thing-that-gurgled", as it was known, didn't work, and the fish felt choked. Sometimes it sucked young fry into itself for its nourishment.

In the winter, the sky froze and the fish were totally isolated from the rest of the Universe. The God figure was not seen at all, but nor were the spear-monsters. The solid sky offered protection as well as detachment.

The plants in the pond were strange life forms. They were useful because they used the fish excrement as food, but that's why the fish thought them odd. They were also useful at making the water more breathable. But they were quiet, they had no worries at all. They were useful for offering hiding places from the aliens. All-in-all, on balance, the plants were nice things, but strange, for the reasons stated before. But, even they were not immune to outside forces. Some of the aliens ate them. Sometimes the Hand-of-God would pull them out of the world.

If, and when, they came back, they usually had received some brutal surgery.

The fish wanted life to be easier. They wanted to have more room to swim. They wanted less danger. They wanted more food. Even though they should have been happy, they felt that life had more to offer. They felt that their God should be more benevolent.

During the summer, the man that the fish thought was a God, sat in a garden chair next to his pond. He watched the fish slowly swimming around. The man was drinking a beer with his friend. They were discussing life and death, as men do when inspired to philosophy by alcohol.

"It is difficult to accept that there is a God." The man said. "Whenever I pray for something that I need, my prayers never seem to be answered. If God existed, surely He would provide everything that I need for a happy life. My car needs upgrading. I want to build a swimming pool before I go on holiday. Why can't He let me have the money I need?"

He opened another bottle and sighed.

"Look at the easy life the fish in my pond have. All of their needs are taken care of and they never thank me for what I do. They don't realise how easy their lives are."

The other man replied.

"Sometimes I think that our understanding of our Creator is like those fish think of you. They can theorise and speculate all they want, but they will never comprehend what really happens in the world outside the pond that they think is their world. How sad it must be to be so restricted in your thinking."

He paused. "Let's have another beer."

5. THE VULTURE'S STORY.

Sitting high on the rocks, the vulture saw the body of the antelope that had been killed by the lion. It could smell its presence as clearly as it could see the source of its next meal.

The bird flapped its wings and then glided to be closer to the corpse. Out of the reach of the lion, it planned its movements for when the big cat had eaten its fill and had withdrawn. Then, it would be in competition with others like itself. Sometimes, there was more danger in being a scavenger than in being a predator.

None of the other animals of the plain liked the vulture. It was seen as ugly and callous. A dealer in death that was too lazy to find its own prey. And it was perceived as ugly because it lacked the magnificent head plumage of the eagles so that it could avoid contamination from the germs that would breed in the blood trapped in its feathers. Its long and gangly legs enabled it to hop around like a dancer to avoid the other maulers at the larder. But those legs made it look comical. Its need to circle over a sick animal whilst waiting for its end to arrive made it seem like an omen of death as it glided on its huge wings.

All in all, the vulture had a poor reputation. There were never witnesses to the care with which it tended to its offspring. There were never observers of the love it shared with its partner. Their offspring and mates never saw them as repulsive.

But the other animals shouted abuse at the vultures whenever they saw them. They called them parasites that lived by celebrating in the death of others. The vultures were hurt by these insults but were never able to defend themselves.

But by now, the antelope was dead and its spirit hovered over its body. Then, the spirit was aware of a voice.

"What would you wish to happen to your body?" it asked. "How would you like your remains to be disposed of now that you have no more use for them?"

The antelope was shocked, but replied quickly. "Please keep the vultures away. I have always hated them. I'd like them to disappear so that my children and grandchildren will be safer."

The voice thought about its reply for a while. "What I will do is show you what the world would be like without vultures."

The spirit of the antelope hovered and watched. The lion had eaten its fill and had wandered away to sleep. Time seemed to accelerate and sped by. The antelope watched as its body rotted and decayed. In the heat of the sun the corpse became contaminated by germs, and was corrupted by infectious organisms.

Disease started to spread outwards. Flies and other insects carried the germs to other creatures that then became sick. When they died their bodies became new breeding grounds for this pestilence.

In time the animals of the plain vanished, including the children and grandchildren of the antelope.

Feeling shocked, the spirit of the antelope gasped. "Does this mean that without the vulture, life would cease. I cannot believe that would happen."

The voice replied slowly. "This was a scenario that was made for you. Within your stomach you had different chemicals and organisms that converted the grass and leaves that you ate into your flesh. That flesh made you and it made your children. The grass became the milk that you gave them to drink and then the food that they needed to grow. Think of the vulture as part of the Earth's digestive system. It converts the old rotting flesh that can cause disease, into manure that the grasses and other plants need to feed on.

In other words, the vulture is the thing that converts your defunct body back into living antelopes in the generations that will follow you. As revolting as you think they are, they and the other scavengers, are essential to the healthy operation of the life of the Earth.

Just because something seems ugly, it does not mean that it has no value. The participants in the performance of life have different faces. Do not assume that those that look like rascals are villains anymore than those that look innocent are angels. Sometimes the things that you should fear most have the sweetest appearance."

The spirit of the antelope was happy now and watched contentedly as the vulture hopped to start the process of renewal, knowing that within an unknown space of time, the antelope would live again through its offspring.

6. THE SALMON'S STORY

It was time to go with the flow. The young salmon had grown big enough to leave the steady pool in the stream and let the current take it to its destiny.

The safety of its birthplace was comfortable. It knew every reed and every pebble that made this part of the river seem so familiar. It had a great number of brothers and sisters as well as cousins and friends, although some disappeared well before their time for them to do so. The young fish was told that they had been eaten by birds and other fish, so it was wary of any other creature that was not a salmon.

But today, the urge to leave became very strong and it moved into the current, and rather than feeding and returning to its customary pool, it carried on downstream, joining many of its friends and relations in this journey.

They called themselves 'The Shoal of Many Parts'. They were not just collections of individuals, they thought of themselves as one big fish.

As they travelled, they found that their rate of growth increased. By the time that they neared the end of the river, they had grown into beautiful, and much bigger individual fish but the numbers had fallen dramatically along the way.

By the time that they had arrived in the sea, the sensation of the change from freshwater to sea-water creatures was strange as their bodies changed to cope with the new environment. But they felt that there had been a metamorphosis from infancy to maturity at that point. They now felt old enough to have wisdom.

In the sea there was an even bigger choice of food, but also a much bigger variety of predators so many more of the 'Big Shoal' were lost.

Swimming towards deeper water, the remaining fish encountered older salmon who were willing to give advice about the better parts of the oceans of the world. They wanted to tell them that were the best feeding grounds, and the safer waters that had fewer hunters.

Some listened and took the advice that they were given. Some listened and ignored it. But others did not listen at all and swam off in search of their own adventures. And so the 'Big Shoal' became three smaller groups of fairly equal size.

The fish in our story was one of those who took the advice of the older salmon and swam and swam for miles and miles in the vast expanse of the oceans of the world. It explored the world and experienced so much. It had used the experiences of others to avoid the most deadly hazards but it also learnt what was safe and what was dangerous from it own experiences. It travelled to where the best feeding grounds were and it enjoyed the company of its remaining companions.

In its travels it sometimes met younger salmon at

the start of their adventures. Remembering the good advice that it was given, it passed on its knowledge and watched how the big shoals divided afterwards.

After a number of years in the oceans, the surviving salmon heard the voice of their ancestors calling them to come home in order to make the next generation. They began swimming home as if they were being carried by a current as strong as that of the river in which they had started their own lives.

After all this time there were still quite a lot of the original group left, but it became smaller by the time they reached the mouth of the river. Predators were aware of the return of the salmon at this time of year, and waited for their bounty.

Swimming in the brackish water as their bodies changed to cope with the fresh water of the river, they reminisced about their times at sea and how they had enjoyed the good times. But they also remembered the times when they had been saddened whenever a member of the group had been lost.

Then a number of salmon from the original 'Shoal of Many Parts' arrived, some looking tired and injured. These were the remnants of the group that listened to the advice of the older fish, but chose to ignore it, at the time. They explained how their numbers had been decimated by predators who would surround them and then break up the shoal, picking off the fish that became vulnerable. The fish decided to recall the advice that they had been given and to act upon it. By the time that they had arrived in safer waters they were a much smaller group, but felt that they had enjoyed a much richer sea life than the first group. By the time that they heard the voice of recall, and had made the journey to the river mouth, they were only about half the number of the first group, but they felt that their lives had been more satisfying.

Then the few remaining salmon from the third shoal, those that had ignored the advice, arrived boasting about the adventures they had experienced. A lot of their number had been eaten, but the survivors had seen parts of the ocean that the others had not. They were the fish that bragged about their strength and their fulfilment.

The huge battle with the river current started soon after this reunion and many salmon were lost between the sea and the pool that they remembered from their earliest moments. Using up the might and muscle that they had developed at sea, they fought against the current and the barriers of waterfalls that they encountered. If they were lucky, they avoided the big furry animals that waited for them if they strayed too close to the banks to find less strong flows.

But a good number of them made it to the spawning grounds, exhausted but able to feel content that they had completed the circle from infancy to a natural end.

Some were rich with experiences, some had encountered more than others, but in the end, as survivors, they would all provide the next stock of adventurers. When that had been accomplished, they knew that this small remainder of the original group would all swim to the Great Ocean to be united with the 'The Shoal of Many Parts', in whichever form that would be.

There they could discuss the merits of embracing risk at the price of danger, or taking the safer options and missing chances. Come what may, there they would be at peace.

7. THE FROGS' LADDER

From the beginning of time, the frogs had wanted to find the ceiling of the world.

The Greatest, Greatest Grandfather, that is the very first frog, set the task, believing that he could reach the ceiling very easily himself, by stretching upwards.

He managed to get a good view, but he was too small to achieve what he wanted.

Perhaps, he thought, my son could reach the sky. So he helped his son to climb onto his shoulders in order to reach higher than he had been able to himself.

The son was unable to reach the objective, but saw more than his father had. He was not grateful because he thought that it was his function in life to progress beyond the feeble foundation that he stood on.

But he never reached the sky.

Perhaps, he thought, my son could reach the sky. So he helped his son to climb onto his shoulders in order to reach higher than he had been able to do himself.

The son was unable to reach the objective, but saw more than his father had. He was not grateful because he thought that it was his function in life to progress beyond the feeble foundation that he stood on.

But he never reached the sky.

The story could, of course go on for ever and ever, but we do not have enough time.

Each generation that stood on the top for a while thought that all the other frogs beneath them had done so for the frog at the peak, until that frog had to allow another to climb onto its own shoulders.

One day a wise bird flew to visit the frog whose turn it was to be at the summit. It laughed at the futility of such a task. All of the frogs in the ladder had missed so much in their search for the unobtainable. The bird told the frog that the sky was so high that it could never be reached. What they had found was ingratitude. They never thanked the frogs below them for their efforts. They had never been grateful to the other frogs in the ladder for their contribution.

The bird told the frog that when something puts others above itself in an effort to help them, the one on top assumes that it is its natural place in life and feels only able to look down on those others that had sacrificed so much.

What all the other frogs should have done was to put their own interests first. When they realised that they would never reach the sky, they should have clambered down to enjoy their lives rather than giving their lives to those who would follow, in the pursuit of the elusive.

"After all," the bird said, "if it were so great up here, why would we birds spend so much time sitting on trees and lakes like the frogs do? Spend your time more wisely. Leave the rat-race to the rats. They deserve it."

With that retort, the bird flew away. The frog at the top started to climb down, slowly. It was polite enough to thank every frog's body on its way, including the pile of crumbled bones at the bottom that were once the Greatest, Greatest Grandfather.

8. THE HAWK'S STORY

When the cage door was left open one day, the hawk sat and looked at the outside world. It was familiar with those big open spaces and the very tall sky because everyday it would be taken from its perch and flown by its owner.

But the hawk had no idea of freedom. It didn't even have a name because it was a tool rather than an individual.

After being taken from its parents as a small chick, it had been raised by its keeper. It had been trained to fly and to hunt for the quarry that it always returned as a demonstration of its reliance upon its owner.

Its duty was to catch two or three rabbits that it then would deliver to its master in return for a small scrap of meat. After its work was done, it was returned to its small cubicle.

Of course, the bird had no concept of being either happy or unhappy because it lacked the experience that allowed it to review its state of emotional well-being. It had its job to do and even felt proud from time to time at the thought that it was providing food and nourishment for its master's family. And after all, in the evening, it would get the entrails of its prey for its supper.

There was a time that the hawk remembered when it had seen a flock of pigeons from its hovering point in the sky. Thinking that they would add variety to its usual routine, it dived at the bird that seemed most isolated from the rest.

Catching it in its talons, the hawk returned it to its master. However, instead of praise the hawk received criticism. What would the man's family do with a pigeon? It was too small to share out and it was difficult to cook with rabbits. The man threw the limp pigeon onto the ground and carried the hawk to another place to go about its task of providing its proper prey.

That evening the hawk became saddened by many things. It was upset that it was not offered the pigeon to eat. It was sad that the pigeon's life had been wasted. Most of all, it was very puzzled at the memory of the sight of a flock of birds. This hawk had always been on its own. Why was it necessary for the pigeons to fly with so many similar others? Who were their masters, and what did they have to catch in order to provide food for those people?

And even on that day that the cage door was left open, the hawk did not have a feeling of liberation. It felt like rejection when its master strutted past the cage, proudly carrying a huge eagle.

The hawk had been aware that there was another bird being trained because it had heard its mewing sounds as well as the whistles from the master; sounds with which it was so familiar.

The master stopped and spoke words that the hawk could not fully understand, but the impression that it had was that the master had trained something bigger and better than itself.

The man had opened the cage door, pushed the eagle towards the hawk, and said, "Within the next hour, you will have the company of this eagle. Then the eagle will kill and eat you. You are no longer needed, and I have no intention of feeding you anymore." The eagle flapped its wings in an attempt to fly and the man was distracted. He walked away but, struggling to control the bigger bird, forgot to close the door properly.

The hawk did not comprehend what had been said, but it felt very uncomfortable. The eagle seemed to evoke a sense of threat. But now it had a choice to make. It could fly away and be on its own or it could stay in the hope that the man would change his mind.

After a while the hawk decided to please its master by taking advantage of the open door in order to fly out to catch food. It soared into the sky and flew to the hillside where he knew its game fed.

It took some time to catch a suitable rabbit. The hawk wanted its gift to be impressive and hunted for the fattest one that it could carry back.

When it returned to its master's house, the hawk flew to its cage. It wanted to leave the rabbit at the door and fly off to catch more. However, the cage door was closed. The eagle was inside, preening itself. As the hawk arrived the eagle made loud threatening noises and flapped its wings to scare the hawk away.

The bird was dejected and did not know what to do. It did not know how to prepare its prey in such a way that the entrails would be exposed. It had no idea that the flesh was the most nutritious part. It pecked away for a while, but left the carcass in the end.

Then, feeling hungry, it flew to a forest on a hill and searched for a tree that had branches that were reminiscent of its cage. It was tired and upset and it needed to sleep, but the night proved to be long and cold. The bird felt so very insecure.

The next morning the hawk took to the sky and returned to its cage in the hope that the door would be open and the eagle gone. The cage was empty, but the door was shut.

In a state of panic, the hawk started to fly towards the rabbit hills to find its master, when suddenly, there was the rush of wind as the eagle lunged at it at great speed, just missing the hawk with its huge claws.

The hawk let out a screech of terror that matched the intensity of the cry of victory from the eagle as they both rolled in a display of acrobatics as the eagle tried to capture the hawk.

Then other shrieks joined the noise, as four other hawks appeared. The frightened bird knew that its death was close. It wanted to give up, to die quickly so it rotated to expose its belly.

As it did so, it could see the other birds mobbing the eagle, whose joy had now become distress. The newly arrived birds indicated that the first hawk should join in, and they all chased the eagle for miles and miles, darting at it now and then to keep it alarmed. The hawk felt elated but did not know why. It was not even sure what the feeling of elation that it experienced was.

And after a good chase the hawks, as one, turned away and flew into a forest where they landed in a row on a big branch.

The eagle, however, was totally lost and it flew away, as its heart instructed, to a mountain a long way from its master's house, to enjoy its own new feeling of release. And, from that point onwards, its natural animosity towards hawks became one of kind regard.

As that first day passed by, the hawks chatted about the fun they had shared until the first hawk realised that it now understood what freedom was. It had been trapped and used for such a long time, just for the benefit of others. Its first experience of liberty had been frightening and potentially deadly. However the world outside the cage was far more fulfilling than the apparent safety that had been its universe before. And the days moved by and the hawk found happiness and fulfilment as it learnt the skills needed for its survival, and the survival of its new family.

The loser in this, of course, was the bird exploiter who had lost both his slaves in one day, by thinking he was being so clever when, in fact, he was being so unkind.

9. THE FLY'S STORY

There had to be a way out! The fly could see where it wanted to fly but there was an invisible something in the way. It had heard about banging heads against brick walls, but this was not brick, nor wood, nor anything that it had any knowledge about.

So it settled on this force field and tried to work out what had happened. Behind it there was the dark space of a room. The where it had landed was not safe, however. Earlier, when it had set down to soak up some sweet white crystals, a rush of wind alerted it to move out of the way of a speeding newspaper. It flew to the safer space it could see in the distance.

Bang! Its head collided with this strange barrier that it could not see, but certainly felt. A little shaken, it buzzed around looking for a way through. It knew there must be one because it could see other flies in the open beyond the veil.

The fly buzzed to the left but found a wooden barrier. It buzzed to the right, to the top, to the bottom. The same wooden fence was there as well. It tried and tried to get through without success.

Then an image of a fly appeared on the other side of the obstruction. The fly was perplexed. There they stood feet to feet, proboscis to proboscis, eye to eye. Neither knew what was happening but both thought that they were looking at themselves and rotated their heads as they puzzled about this strange phenomenon.

When they realised that they were two different flies that were separated by this puzzling screen, they both asked each other, in that strange foot waggling way of speech that they have, how did they progress to the other side. The new fly could see the sugar in the distance and wanted its share. The fly on the inside wanted to get out, however. It needed to be away from rolled up newspapers.

So they both struggled. One wanting to get in, the other wanting to escape.

Then there was a mighty 'thwack!'.

The new fly was frightened away by the noise and vibration. The first fly was squashed on the window. The new fly had moved back some distance but returned to see what had happened to its new friend. It looked bigger somehow. All of it touched the barrier. It was still. It could not speak.

The new fly moved away from the glass in shock. When it returned it somehow passed through the force field. In actual fact it had found the gap of the open window.

Feeling pleased with itself it flew to the sugar bowl, it forgot about its unfortunate new acquaintance. As it fed on the sweetness, it was surprised when it realised that in order to get through the obstacle, it had to fly away from it and return from a new angle.

This, perhaps, was a revelation. When confronted by a problem, move away, think, and return with a different line of approach. This way, even the invisible barriers and obstacle may be overcome.

It knew that one of the great dangers for flies is the barely visible spiders' web. Because it looks flimsy there is the temptation to fly through it rather than around. This fly had lost a lot of its friends in this way. They were unable to see the danger in those things that looked safe. The things that were obviously dangerous such as walls could be avoided or landed on.

The hazards that were the most deadly involved those things that seemed to be safe, like the newly found, but not seen obstacle, and cobwebs that did not show their ability to trap.

It knew that there are risks in the easy and sweet ways. As the fly became preoccupied with its sucking in of the sweetness of the sugar, it did not notice the rolled-up newspaper starting its descent.

10. THE WEB

What a mess!

The web that the spider was spinning seemed tangled, knotted and generally awful. The other spiders laughed. The flies even chuckled on their way past, and even carried on smiling if they got caught in the meshes of the other spiders' nets, until their laughter turned to tears.

Of course, it was no joke. This poor spider's life was like its attempts at web making. It had tried so hard to weave its existence into some sort of order. No matter what it did, something seemed to go wrong. A strand would break, or a twig that the mainstay was attached to, snapped off. It appeared to be disaster at every stage. It was as if the word 'snag' had been invented to describe this spider's attempts at progress.

Its relationships were also complex and disastrous. Its future was hard to predict, its hopes had so little chance of becoming reality. It was as if the problems it had experienced in its life were being drawn into the frustrations in its creation of its web.

The spider wanted to give up. It wanted to consume the gossamer and start all over again. It was hungry and insecure. It felt so vulnerable to the birds and other creatures that wanted to eat it. It was panicky and distressed.

Out of a sense of surrender, it decided to let fate and coincidence play their parts in the development of the web. The spider wanted it to reflect the mess in its life, to represent the chaos that reigned. All through that night it spun and spun. It wove and wove. Blindly, it continued, with no idea of what the outcome would be. The release of the strands from its glands was like the pouring of emotions from its heart.

The following morning, the outcome looked so ridiculous to the other spiders. Instead of the square mesh that they made, this web radiated outwards into a circle with concentric circles. It did look strangely beautiful, however, with the early morning light shining on the droplets of dew that had condensed onto it. The spider felt proud of its efforts but ashamed of the results.

When the other spiders saw the cobweb, they laughed even more loudly than ever before. "Where are the vertical and horizontal lines?" They goaded. "Where are the big knots where the strands meet?" The spider sat in the middle of its web and wept tears that obscured the drops of dew.

Then a big juicy fly flew into the neighbourhood. It landed on one of the square webs, but before it was caught, it slipped through the net and flew on, giggling loudly. This was a smug fly! Some of them were, back then!

It did the same to the other spiders, but when it saw the circular web, it laughed almost hysterically. It flew deliberately into it, became entangled, and before it knew what happened, the spider ran along one of the spokes and pounced onto it. The spider ate the hearty meal that it needed so desperately.

The other spiders gasped in amazement, but they put it down to luck. However their laughter was noticeably quieter than before! They watched closely as events unravelled.

The days went by. The spider with the round cobweb caught more and more food, while the others started to go hungry. They had all stopped laughing except for the spider that had produced the new style of web. Every time a fly became entangled, the spider let out chuckles and chortles, not of derision for the others, but of contentment for itself.

With a sense of hopelessness, the other spiders arranged a meeting with the successful one. They studied the structure of the web. They realised that strength came from a circle rather than a square. They saw that the radiating strands gave faster access to the entrapped prey. They came to view the assumed chaos as a different kind of order. They began to admire the first spider for its genius in being able to disregard the past constraints of convention in order to progress way beyond the limitations of what was customary.

They recognised that just because something seems tangled and hopeless, it does not mean that the results will be less worthwhile than they would with something that appears to be simpler, but logical and planned. The mess that the spider's life seemed to be in, actually led to great success and admiration.

Sometimes, it seems, the mess that life appears to be in, can lead to something that is more useful and valuable than what is, apparently, traditional and straightforward.

The spider was now surrounded by others who had respect and admiration for its creativity and nerve. Those other spiders started to recycle their old gossamer, and copied the design of that spider who used to be anxious and disturbed, but was now at peace.

As did all of the other spiders of the world, in due course, as you can see early in the morning of every day.

HUMAN NATURE

11. REJECTION

The man sat at the top of a cliff and thought about how his marriage had ended. His wife had left him without warning so that she could be on her own.

Many years before, when his wife's father had first learnt that he was going to have a child, he was delighted. He and his wife had been trying for a long time without success.

When the girl was born he was disappointed that he had not fathered a son, but he was happy enough. Having a son would show the world that he was a real man, a man strong enough to sire strong men like himself, but having a daughter proved he was capable of breeding. When his daughter was growing up she shared love with her father, she felt at the top of his mountain. As years went by, and as no other children were forthcoming, he was content to allow her to be the most important thing in his life.

However, when the girl was seven, her wife became pregnant again. The family was delighted. The girl would have a playmate, somebody to share her young world with, after all this time.

When the man's son was born, he was so happy. He had a son and heir, he had real proof of his masculinity.

The girl felt a little rejected because so much attention was now paid to her brother, but when she tried to play with him she was told to leave him alone. He was the apple of her father's eye. The girl had fallen off his mountain.

She became quiet, and she cried a lot. She felt hurt. She wanted to be happy, loving and expressive but was told to be quiet or she would wake the baby. Her father kept shouting at her. He made all sorts of threats about what would happen if she went near his precious son.

She hid herself away and just wanted to be alone. She thought that she had a friend to play with at last, but she was not allowed to get anywhere near him. Her father was so aggressively offensive.

When the girl grew up she met a man whom she loved. They married and after a few years, they had a son. The woman knew what to do, she had learnt well as a child. She gave all her love to her son at the expense of her husband. Her son was hers. Her son would love her forever. She would never be rejected again.

Now, the woman's husband understood what was happening. He knew how aggressive his father-in-law was, and could see how he had built fear of rejection into his daughter's character. He realised that he was married to a woman who wanted to reject the man who loved her, the man who had built his world around her, before she was rejected by him. She was getting older, and she felt less attractive, even though her husband thought that she was still the most beautiful woman in the Universe. She felt that her husband's feelings of hurt at her rejection of him, were his way of showing his disapproval of her. So she felt that he was beginning to discard her. This was not so.

He realised that the crisis point in the marriage had been after his wife had travelled to her brother's village with her parents for her brother's wedding. Before the trip, his wife had been very ill and had recuperated with her parents where her father had treated her as a little girl for the first time in many years.

She felt, once again, as she had when she was the only child. Her father cared for her, and he had looked after her. Then, at her brother's wedding, she had been pushed aside as her brother became the centre of attention, once again, and she felt resentful.

Out of a sense of family loyalty, she felt that she could not blame her ageing father, and she needed somebody younger, somebody at the age of her father when her brother had arrived, to push those feelings of rejection onto. So, her husband became the recipient, the victim.

He opened his eyes and realised that his wife had lived a life where she felt that anything that she became strongly attached to, would reject her. So she had developed a rule of 'reject before being rejected'. And, in this way she thought that she would never be hurt again.

12. POISONING THE WELL

The desert was hot, very hot. As the sun rose higher in the sky, the pleasure that is usually felt from warmth, became an intense pain.

As the man reached the well, he was near exhaustion. He was very dry. The water was cool and clean from the bucket that he had raised. He sat next to the stone surround while he slaked his thirst.

The man was bitter about his experiences. He had fought with the chief of his village after the chief had said something that the man had objected to. So he had left his home, vowing never to return.

He took a big bag of poison with him in order to avoid being followed. Every time that he came to one of the few wells in the desert, he drank, filled his bottles, put poison into the bucket and continued on his way. In that way he sought revenge by hurting the other villagers.

The desert was as big as the man's sense of loneliness and isolation. After a long time he reached the foothills of the mountains where he moved into a new village. He was proud that he had poisoned every well between this new place and his village. He could never be followed. He was also proud that he had achieved a new life with new people.

When the earthquake happened it was without warning. The village was destroyed and a huge canyon appeared. His new friends were gone and he was on his own again. There was no food and no water. He had no choice but to move into the desert.

The desert was hot, very hot. As the sun rose higher in the sky, the pleasure that is usually felt from warmth, became an intense pain.

As the man reached the well, he was near exhaustion. He was very dry. The water was cool and clean from the bucket that he had raised. He sat next to the stone surround while he slaked his thirst.

And so, his promise that he would never return to his village was kept.

13. THE PRECIOUS VASE

The vase had been given to the woman by her grandmother. It was worth a great deal, not just for its material value, but more for the sentiments that it contained.

The woman had loved her grandmother very much, although she had been very strict with her when she was growing up. The constraints placed upon her as a child had led her to hold any annoyance that she felt until it had become intense anger. This was usually vented upon her husband.

Her husband was a caring man who had become familiar with her outbreaks of temper. However, her foul tantrums had put a strain on their marriage, but he understood to an extent.

Nevertheless, he was getting to the point when he was not willing to take very much more and he approached his wife with the proposal that she should seek some help.

She erupted. She exploded. She called him all the horrible names that she could, and then invented more to insult him with.

She picked up a jug from the far side of the room and threw it at him. He ducked and it whistled past his ear to smash against the wall. Next, she threw a plate, and then a cup. She looked at the vase but left it in its place, opting for a bowl that his mother had given them, instead. Her destructive spell ended as she stormed out of the house to get away from her man.

She walked deep into the forest and sat by a small stream, allowing her tears to join the flow.

Of course she loved her husband. He was the most precious thing in her life. She wondered why she hurt him so much. She questioned why she treated him the way she did. She had no idea why she lacked the control necessary to stop her outbursts.

As she pondered, she seemed to hear the babbling of the stream as a voice that was talking to her.

"You do have control, my dear." The voice was uncannily like her grandmother's. "When you were throwing things like the jug, the cup, the plate and your tantrums, you decided not to throw the vase that I gave to you. Something made you think about, and to evaluate, the damage that you might do.

That is your control. You have it. Isn't it strange that you value the vase more highly than your relationship with your husband? Do you think that he only married you so that he could soak up all of the childhood anguish that you brought with you?

If you break the vase, then you can shed a tear, then buy a new one. If you break your husband, then you have lost far more. You will have lost something that you will be unable to replace, because if you did find a new man, you would treat him in the same way.

Use the control that you used with the vase to protect, love and care for the thing in your life that far more value than a piece of clay."

The woman was ware of footsteps behind her. It was her husband who had come to make sure that she was alright.

He said, "I am sorry that I upset you. I am sorry that I made you lose your temper."

The woman started to sob. She reached out to hug this precious man and said. "I have lost my temper. I have lost it for evermore. Please forgive me for the way I used to be."

They walked back to their home, hand-in-hand, like young lovers once again.

14. THE FISHERMAN'S STORY

There was once a fisherman who was very proud of his fine canoe. He had built it and had improved it for many years. He was a proud man who was very contented with his way of life. He knew no other and did not wish for anything else.

One day, during his search for fish, his canoe hit a big rock in the rapids. The boat was damaged and this caused him great concern, but he was able to continue. He was sure that once it had been repaired, there would be no more problems. He continued to paddle along, confident that he would complete his journey.

However, a little further downstream the fisherman was caught in a sudden and bad-tempered storm. The canoe was damaged so badly that he was flung into the water.

The boat hit more rocks and was smashed into pieces. He loved his craft and felt so sad. It was cold in the water and the current was strong. It was dark and misty by now. He could not see where he was or where he should go. He thrashed about in the river, desperately looking for a sign of hope. He was very frightened.

Then he saw a part of his beloved canoe. He clung to it so tightly. His hands turned white, and then blue with the cold. Now he noticed that it had become quiet around him as he drifted helplessly, not knowing what his fate would be.

Looking at this last part of his precious vessel, he began to blame himself for this disaster. If only he had paid more attention to his course, if only he had stopped to mend the first damage. If only! He was filled with so much pain and sadness. So much self-reproach. He was grief stricken. He had so loved his boat.

Suddenly, out of the darkness, he heard a voice calling to him. He shouted back to let her know where he was. The voice told him that rescue was at hand, it tried to reassure him, to let him know that he would be alright.

Then this other canoe pulled alongside and a hand reached out to help him. The fisherman was so scared, however. He was afraid to let go of this last piece of his life, but he knew that if he did not let go, he would drift on and on until he was crushed by the great waterfall further on downstream.

15. SURFING LIFE

The man ran to the sea carrying his surfboard. He swam hard to push his way through the breakers until he was ready to turn. He climbed on and allowed the energy, held in the water, to propel him back towards the beach.

He had found the swim out to his turning point very tiring. It reminded him of when he was young and he had to pull his sledge to the top of the hill before he could enjoy the ride back down. He had to work against gravity before he could use it.

He returned to his towel on the beach and mused. He thought about his life. He had worked long and hard to save the money for this short holiday in the sun by the sea. His break from his work and his wife. The comparison to surfing, sledding and playing as a child to his continuing slog of using his energies over a long period of time to gain a short burst of pleasure ran through his mind.

All of his life seemed to be that way. He compared the battery driven toys of his children to the clockwork ones of his earlier days. He felt like those clockwork mechanisms where you had to provide energy to what was, in reality, an energy storage system that slowly released it. For clocks that was. However, most of his toys, like his happiness, spilled that power all too readily, into a rush, before becoming motionless.

As he watched the water, he saw a wind-surfer skipping over the waves. He realised that the man riding the board was using the energy of the breeze to give himself pleasure. There was no effort in swimming against the waves, no climbing to a peak before slipping down. He realised that some people had found an easier path to walk than the one that he had stumbled upon. Maybe he needed a way to find a source of energy that he did not have to provide in the first place. Perhaps, in his life, he should find a breeze rather than a flow that pushed against him. He should be going with the flow: surviving, flourishing, and prospering.

He knew that the small creatures which inhabited the rock pools fed on whatever was washed near them when the tide was coming in, and out. They remained in a static place and let the energy of the sea bring food to them. Perhaps, he thought, he should open a shop! He chuckled to himself. No! That would tie him to a place. The shrimps and shellfish saw very little of the world, and being fixed in a small pool made them prey as well as predators in the food chain. He was not a retailer, that was for sure!

However, his life was a bit like that now. He was like the sledge and the surfboards. He was used by somebody else in order to give pleasure and profit. His boss was the rider, the sailor, who used him. But he, as the used, was the vehicle that was dispensable. He could be broken and smashed by somebody else and then replaced so easily.

His wife seemed to be the same as his boss. She enjoyed the benefits of his pay cheque but showed little gratitude for what he had to do in order to earn it. She had threatened him with divorce because he had become so stressed that he was not able to be jolly and cheerful all the time. It was as if he was expected to be the primeval hunter by day and the court jester in the evening and the perfect lover by night. As a result he felt as replaceable in his marriage as he did in his job.

"In short," he mumbled to himself, "I pull the sledge to the top of the hill, and my boss enjoys the ride down. I swim the surfboard out to the big rollers and my wife surfs back in. I am so sick and tired of all this. I need a sign, symbol or a direction to be given to me."

Like a sulking child he slumped back onto his towel. He sat up a little and stared around him, desperately looking for his portent. He saw nothing that was different. Nothing jumped into his line of vision. No words or pictures presented themselves. Disappointed he got up, collected his surfboard and returned to the small hotel he was staying in.

Later, in the evening, his wife telephoned him to tell him that his boss had called. There was a problem at work and he needed to contact the office as soon as possible. She made some small talk and hung up. He knew that she was irritated because he had taken his week's holiday without her. She did not realise how much he needed to get away from the pressures that were squeezing the life from him.

He made his way to a bar that sat in the horseshoe shaped harbour of the town. He ate some pizza, drank some beer and started to play the old pinball machine that stood in a corner. At least he would clear his mind of his worries for a while by absorbing himself in something of no consequence.

He had enjoyed playing the machines when younger, and as everybody does, he flipped the flippers with great gusto as if flying a fighter plane in combat.

He shot the first steel ball into the field of play and watched it collide with, and bounce off, the domes that gave speed and momentum back to the ball. He heard the chattering and clinking of the score counter making harmonies with the tic-tic-tic noises of the flippers.

He flicked the ball higher back up into the field of play and watched it gently roll into an obstacle that shot it down to the right flipper. Back up again. The game lasted for quite a few minutes until he missed the ball as it shot down into the unreachable gully that took it away.

He shot another ball into play, and partly distracted by a pretty woman who walked in on her own, he just seemed to watch the ball rise up the table and fade down into the chasm of failure at the bottom of the table.

The woman was joined by her husband after parking their car and the man walked back to his hotel. He thought about the day and the evening as he drank another beer.

The pinball table held his thoughts. He felt more like the ball whose destiny was held by randomness and the direction of outside forces. He was pushed and flicked without any say in what was happening.

The ball was him. He was inside the ball, passive and helpless. Moved by outside events and forces. He wanted to be the player. The person who, although having to react to capricious happenings, had the influence to change the flow of those events. He could keep the ball in play for longer; he could score more with a deft flick of his fingers. He needed to control his direction within the randomness of his fate.

Perhaps this was the input that he needed. He knew that he was stressed, control had been outside himself. He was the controlled rather than the controller. He did not want to manipulate his wife or his boss. He did not them to become the globes in his pinball machine. What he wanted and needed was for them to stop playing him.

Resolved to changing his life, he woke the following morning and took his surfboard to the equipment shop. He exchanged it for a sailboard and booked some instruction. Although transparent as a symbol, this was the sign that he needed; the achievement of his badge of control.

He would go with the flow of his own destiny rather than be caught up in the tides and currents of others like a piece of flotsam.

Later that day he telephoned his boss. He told him firmly that he would deal with any problems when he returned to work. He told his boss that as he was senior to himself, then he boss should be fully capable of handling any crisis without having to interrupt his holiday.

And as for his wife...he started to plan his future so that they would be happy together or he would find happiness for himself. He was no longer a pawn in a game, he was starting to live rather than existing to survive.

Although a sailor is unable change the direction of the wind, he is able to change the course of his craft.

With a flicker of hope shining through his worry, he started to make his way to his first wind-surfing lesson.

16. WHO OR WHAT?

It walked into the village one day in the Spring of that year. Nobody knew what it was, but they needed to know.

It was human, like they were, but it was different. It looked taller than most. It appeared to be stronger than most. The strange thing about this strange thing was its skin. Rather than being the same as the villagers, the skin of this thing was covered in black and white chequers. The local people had a tanned skin that shone with sweat in the heat of the day, but blended with the darkness of the sky at night.

The new thing walked to the village centre and asked a tribal elder if he could drink from the well. The old man told the thing that he was not welcome and should leave. The new arrival turned to walk away.

"What are you?" the old man asked him.

The thing turned back and said, "My name is Tottali. That is who I am."

The old man looked at him and said, "I asked you what you are, not who are you. Learn to listen or do you come from a type that is so stupid that you cannot understand simple words? Leave our water alone. We do not want to be contaminated by outsiders. Go, because we do not want strange breeds around these parts." The old man spat in Tottali's face, called him a 'rengo', the worst insult that these people had. He then turned his back and walked to the meeting place nearby.

The old man called out for the other elders to join him to discuss this disturbing development.

Meanwhile, Tottali walked away into the dry grasslands that surrounded the village.

When the elders met they discussed this new arrival. They did not like him. They saw him as a danger. He was big and strong, they were told. He posed a threat to this little community. He would kill and eat the children because he was so primitive. He would probably steal their food and valuables. He would almost certainly rape the women of the village.

They knew all of this because the old man had told them how he looked and how he had been unable to use even simple words. Despite the fact that Tottali had only been seen by one man, the others readily hated him because he was so obviously different. They wanted to hunt him down and kill him as they would a lion.

The children were told that if this thing appeared they should hide and then run back to tell the trackers and hunters where it had been seen.

A week went by and the disquiet that the thing had caused started to quieten down until the villagers were informed that one of the children was missing. The trackers and hunters were sent out to find him, knowing that he had been taken by the strange thing. After all, the old man now told his people that the thing had made a threat of revenge after he had told the thing to stop trying to urinate in the well.

Way out in the bush they found spots of blood and followed the spoor of the chequered thing. They wondered why it had not eaten the boy where it had killed him, but they knew that it was primitive and, therefore thought in an odd way.

Late in the day Tottali was found at a watering hole. They boy was lying on the ground. There was blood on his head. The thing was kneeling over him with a knife.

Three spears hit the thing simultaneously. He did not die but collapsed to the ground silently.

The boy screamed. He told the hunters that he had become lost whilst hunting rabbits, and had found this place. He had been drinking by this watering hole earlier in the day when he had been attacked by a large wild dog. The blood on his head came from the wounds inflicted by its teeth.

He had been rescued by the chequered thing that had suffered many injuries as a result.

The hunters asked about the trail of blood that they had followed and the boy showed them the body of a rabbit he had caught.

The men removed the spears and staunched the bleeding from the holes in the thing's flesh. They picked up the boy and started to carry him back to the village. They left Tottali by the water because they did not know what he was and were afraid to take him back as well.

The story was well told when the men returned with the boy. The village chief was grateful for the thing saving his grandson's life and instructed the hunters to find it and bring it to the village. He was very angry that they had left it behind to perish.

A day later the men brought the chequered thing back and it was placed on a grass bed in the communal place. Men and women tended the thing and as it got better and talked more they realised that this thing was really a person. He was different to look at but under the patterned skin he was the same as them.

The boy who he had saved visited him often and they exchanged stories. This was a good experience for both of them. They had different backgrounds but the stories were similar in that they talked about life and nature, kindness and cruelty, dreams and realities.

When Tottali was able to walk, he busied himself by helping the villagers. He told the hunters about the techniques his people had used and they learnt some new skills. This made the men who had hurt him feel that there was neither anger nor resentment.

After a few months the villagers came to understand that this man was a man with a different skin but he was no threat or danger. He ate no children, raped no women. He was just like them and they realised that they were just like him.

The old man who had spread the evil and nasty stories was treated with a polite contempt. Eventually he found the need to apologise. After he had done so, he chatted with Tottali for many hours. He explained that not only did he realise that the way to view life was to consider who they were rather than what they were. Even the dogs that lived in the village had names. The animals that lived in the bush lands were called by their 'what' names such as lions or antelopes. However, the things that we should be close to were called by their 'who' names. This signified that we had an understanding of the inner nature and personality of the person or animal.

This was, perhaps, the essence of understanding how we should relate to others. We should know who the person is before we form an opinion. To decide upon the nature of a person by quickly giving a superficial description of what they are leads to bigotry and prejudice. The old man had been guilty of that, but had learnt that change is necessary, even in a person who seemed to be fixed in his thinking.

Tottali was nearly healed and decided to return to his home. He said his farewells and started on his way.

He walked out of the village one day in the Autumn of that year. Everybody knew who he was, and were glad that they did.

17. THE THIRD EYE

When humankind was first born, it had horns, big claws and almost impenetrable skin.

Because we had so much protection, however, we became cruel. When people saw other forms of life, they would, very often, kill for fun. Even plants would be ripped from the ground and tossed aside for no reason at all. Men were immune to danger and no other animal could prey on them.

Just to prove how mighty they thought they were, men killed the huge, but gentle, elephants and rhinoceroses for fun. They never ate the flesh but left the flesh to rot in the sun.

The Gods were worried by this creature that claimed dominance over all life on Earth. They met, conversed and decided that the horns of men should be removed and given to the elephants and rhinos for their protection. But nothing changed. Mankind still killed the giants and used their horns and tusks to decorate their caves.

So the Gods met again and decided that the thick skins of men should be removed and given to the elephants and rhinoceroses to protect them from those who had hunted them so needlessly. So mankind was skinned, and still walks naked to this very day.

This eased the problem for the elephants and rhinos because the men were more vulnerable without their armoured skins and horns, and the gentle giants more able to defend themselves.

Because of this, men turned to the inedible big cats for their fun. They used their skins to keep them warm because, being exposed without hide or fur, they felt cold.

So the Gods met again and decided to give the claws of men to the big cats. This changed the balance for a while. Some men were even killed and eaten by lions. Now mankind was the prey rather than the predator. Other animals would creep up behind them and grab them by the scruffs of their necks.

It was then that the Gods thought that they had, perhaps, gone a little too far. They knew that the decisions they had made to remove the offensive and defensive weapons of men were to prevent other species from being wiped out. Now there was the possibility that man would be eliminated instead.

The Gods decided to give men the ability to think in a creative way in order to protect themselves. They also gave men an extra eye. The two he already had were located in the predatory position at the front of the face. The new, third, eye was located at the back of the head so that men could see other creatures that were stalking them.

Men were able to survive in this way but the great streak of cruelty still remained. Whereas some men used their ability to create in helping the

Earth and its inhabitants, others set about making new claws for themselves, calling them knives. Those men then set about making new horns for themselves and called them spears. They used the tough hides from the animals they killed with their new weapons to make shields to replace their thick skins.

Once again the Gods were shocked and disappointed. They had to redress the balance. They turned the third eye inwards so that men could not see dangers from behind. Instead the Gods wanted them to look inside their own minds to see the perils from the biggest threat to life on the Earth; themselves. To this very day we can feel where that eye used to be at the backs of our heads.

Feeling invulnerable once again, the men wanted to punish the Gods for what they had done. Over time they developed their weapons and defences through a game they called 'war'. They killed each other needlessly. They killed animals and plants unnecessarily, including the elimination of whole species and massive forests.

Even though humans were given the facility to view the cruelty within with that inward-facing eye. And to this very day we all know those people who are unable to see with that third eye that we all possess. Cruelty is still the possession of humans.

However, one day soon, the Gods will meet again to decide the next step that they will take.

18. MAGIC

Abracadabra! Nothing happened. Abracadabra! Nothing happened again.

Jeme, the selfish man was disappointed but deep down inside, by now, he had expected nothing to happen. He had read many books on how the universe works, how to reach his destiny, how to influence others, and the secrets of religion and magic. But nothing seemed to work.

He had bought magic wands, drums, talismen and lucky charms. He had meditated, contemplated, observed and considered. However, he was still powerless in his attempts to get what he wanted.

He had repeated a variety of incantations, wishes, spells and curses. He had lit incense sticks and candles.

He had consulted priests, gurus and charlatans. He had sat in stone circles, he had read his horoscopes.

He had consulted ancient works of wisdom.

He had been seen by palm readers, card readers and people who claimed to talk to the dead.

Everything that was tried, failed. Of course, by now, he was frustrated, bewildered and defeated by the world and the people outside of himself. He could not see his future, he could not control his fate, destiny or fortune.

In short, he felt just like everybody else. He wanted to be better than that! He felt that he deserved better than to be so ordinary.

However, he liked beggars and paupers because they made him feel better about himself. He could show them the money he carried and watch the look of sadness in their faces as he walked away with his assets intact.

He also enjoyed selling his impotent tools of magic to others who were desperate to improve their lives, although he usually lost money in the process. His satisfaction came, in part, from proving the items to be powerless. He had the first attempt at extracting their sorcery.

There was one transaction of which he was very proud. He had made a profit by selling an old carved oak staff to a man who could not afford it. Jeme had extracted the last piece of money that his customer had possessed. Jeme had bought the staff from somebody who told him that he could make imperfect things work and could bring huge rewards. Like everything else he had purchased, it had not worked at all. But the day that he sold the staff at a financial gain was one of his, very few, happy days.

Although Datu, the man who bought the staff was very poor in money, he was in fact, very rich in his heart. He had seen a young boy who was unable to walk. His legs had been broken when very small and had set in such a crooked way that he was unable to stand. The kind man had bought the staff to make a pair of crutches rather than to make spells. After he had fashioned them into two sturdy sticks, he gave them to the young man, expecting nothing, not even thanks, for them.

The young man practised with them until he was able to move as if he had not been damaged. Strangely, the staff had made imperfect things work.

Unbeknown to Datu, his act of unselfish generosity had been witnessed by a friend of the richest man in those parts. When the rich man heard what had happened, he was so touched in his heart that he gave some land and buildings to the kind man. The rich man knew that having a kind neighbour would be safer than having a part of his land occupied by a greedy person. He also arranged for him to receive some money to ensure that the kind man would not have to compete with his own businesses.

Well Datu, not content with these gifts, converted his building into a sanctuary for the unfortunate people of the area. He helped them to walk again. He helped them to learn trades. He gave hope to the hopeless and joy to the miserable.

When he heard about this the rich man was so happy because his wealth was bringing happiness to many people as well as himself. He gave more and more money, buildings and land to Datu to expand his work. People from all over the land learnt what was happening. The trades of the rich man flourished because other traders knew that this man must be trustworthy. In this strange way, the rich man became very happy as well as rich. He was using his wealth to create the thing that could not be bought, peace of mind. Datu developed his work to include as many of the very many unfortunate people of the land that it was possible to help.

One day Jeme, the selfish man, saw Datu with a man walking on crutches. He recognised that they were made from the staff because he saw the intricate carvings that had been made for such a magical wand.

He followed them back to the settlement and asked to meet the kind man. Datu felt that he had met this man before and felt uncomfortable, somehow. He did not know why.

At that point, the man who had been the young man, walked in on his crutches. He told Datu that he was the person who had sold him the staff. He then said that as it had brought so much good fortune the kind man should share some of the money that he had made with himself. After all, he said, he was the man who had promised him good fortune from the magical staff. He even offered to sell him some more instruments to make far more money. Datu looked at him, and smiled in a kind way.

He replied in soft tones. He told Jeme that the staff was, indeed, a strong and powerful thing. He explained how it had helped a young man to walk again. He described how that act of kindness had resulted in the growth of kindness and care for others.

The selfish man was perplexed and asked the kind man which magic words and spells he had used. He begged to know which rituals were performed to empower the staff to bring so much good fortune. He wanted to find out how he could bring such good fortune upon himself.

Datu told the man to give all his money to the poorest man he could find before the sun set on the following day. After that he should return to be told the magic words that should be spoken to bring good luck.

The selfish man left, disgruntled and cursing under his breath. He had tried all sorts of things, but he could never bring himself to the point of foolish generosity. And so, he never returned. He was too frightened that the magic phrase would not work for him. He was too worried that he would lose the little he had. The thought that his money should be given to the beggars and luckless was too much for him to consider.

After Jeme, the selfish man, had failed to come back, the young man looked at the Datu, the kind man and told him that he knew what the magic words were.

Without waiting for a prompt to answer he said, "Here, have what I have. You need it more than I do." The young man paused and then added; "I know those words because they were the ones you said to me when you gave me my crutches."

The kind man smiled and replied. "Those words have much greater magic in them than anything else. The selfish man ends up with only himself as his friend. I am blessed with being a channel of plenty rather than its container. Magic is based on intention rather than the end."

The young man saw a boy with broken legs being carried in by his father. As he handed his crutches to the boy he said, "Here, have what I have. You need it more than I do." The smile on his face was as bright as the sun in the summertime.

19. THE SCAPEGOAT'S STORY

Way back in time the Scapegoats were big and cuddly animals. They had broad backs and thick skins. They had been specially bred to share the problems of people, which they did with a great sense of pleasure.

However, over time they had been burdened with the task of taking the responsibility and blame for any failings that became apparent in any person's life. Every family had one and, very often, different people would use the same one whenever they felt like it.

Then, one day the Great Creator felt angry at the abuse of these noble creatures and decided to give them liberty. It was decided that they would be reassigned to a much happier life and a plan was devised.

Suddenly, a disease spread through the species which, whilst giving outward signs of pain and terror, actually gave great pleasure as they transformed into their new structures.

So what mankind saw as their extinction was, in fact, the moment of freedom when the Scapegoats were re-created as albatrosses where the breezes would support them effortlessly as they explored the joys of life, rather than its misery.

Naturally, most of humankind decided that this epidemic must have been, after all, the Scapegoat's own fault, so they must have deserved their fate. But the need to give others the blame still remained, and those caring people, who had sympathy for the vanished creatures, very naturally became their substitutes. Although there was nothing different about them when they were born, any weakness that was shown enabled them to be crafted and developed much more easily, by the selfish people, than the years of breeding that would have been necessary to develop a new creature like the original Scapegoats.

Things, or people to blame, were felt to be so essential for a happy life. For example, if the hunt was bad, the men had somebody to rebuke. If a woman felt that her marriage was not working, she could chastise her human Scapegoat.

People could invent all sorts of stories about the reasons for their misery, and assign them to one person. After shifting accountability, they would always feel so much better.

However, the replacements for the Scapegoats had not been bred for the job. Their backs were often not broad enough, nor their skins thick enough to be able to carry the load. Unlike the big creatures before them, they would break down and suffer from their inflicted misery without help. The Blamers would assume that their miserable state was their own failing anyway, so they were shown no sympathy.

The Great Creator was disappointed with this state of affairs and pondered long and hard about what the solution should be. It had to different to the 'plague of delight' that had liberated the first Scapegoats.

Specific elements of a society could not be made immune, and it was not possible to relieve the Blamers of their lack of responsibility for their own actions. That was a self-inflicted condition that came from a lack of care and an abundance of selfishness.

So this time, a two-phase plan came into effect. A 'plague of separation' was spread whereby people could only be with others like themselves.

So, male Blamers would get together to complain about how bad their lives had been because of the women in their lives. Female Blamers, of course, would condemn the men. And so on.

But, after the separation of the two types, the human Scapegoats had nobody to blame them for anything, so they started to feel unwanted.

And so it happened that after a while, when the human Scapegoats had all left to be together, the Blamers had nobody to blame for what was going wrong with their lives so they had to start blaming each other.

But, as the Blamers thought themselves to be perfect, wars broke out. Many people were destroyed and the population declined. Seeing this devastation, they had no option but to take the blame upon themselves for so much chaos in the

World, because nobody else would accept it, and they had to blame somebody.

Meanwhile, the human Scapegoats, being innocent of the bloodshed, started to blame the Blamers for the terrible desolation that now pervaded the Earth.

As planned, after a number of years, the balance between self-accountability and the need to blame those who really were at fault, was achieved in both societies. Now all the people were able to come back together.

People had learnt to accept responsibility for their own mistakes and to work for self-improvement. The Blamers learnt to stop blaming others for the mistakes that they had made themselves. And the Scapegoats learnt to reject any disapproval if they were, in fact, free of error.

At last, everybody was able to offer constructive advice if requested, and they all learnt to withhold unnecessary criticism of others.

But, while the albatrosses lived their lives in peace, the humans started to revert to their old ways.

And who can we blame for that?

NATURE'S NATURE

20. THE MOOD RAINBOW

The boy sat with his grandfather by the bank of a river. The sky became dark as the rain started in the distance.

As a rainbow appeared the boy asked the old man to help him to find the pot of gold that would be at its end. The man told the boy that the real treasure existed in the story that the rainbow could tell.

He began to explain.

"The rainbow is made from the splitting of perfect light. Raindrops act as small prisms to split pure light into its different parts. But as the colours show themselves when light passes through from the bright side, the colours cannot be seen on the dark side. Those colours of the rainbow, when mixed as paints, make the opposite, they make gloom and darkness.

The moods of people are like the colours of the rainbow. Sometimes those moods make perfection, sometimes they make the opposite.

Take red for example. It represents the energy of strong action whether good or bad. It is the colour of fire which helps to manufacture or to destroy.

In its pure form red is for the action needed for protection, as happened in mans' early times to fend off predators.

It is the energy that is used to fight obstacles in the way of progress.

It is also an expression of determination.

However, negative red force is used for anger, for rage, for revenge and the pointless destruction of objects, people and relationships.

Orange is the colour of the sunrise and the birth of new days. Some days are good, some are bad. Just as the birth of most people is good news, but the birth of dictators and tyrants is not.

And yellow is the colour of the sun. It represents light, brightness and hope in its perfect form. It is about hope and positive attitudes.

In its hostile form it is the colour of a barren and empty desert that poses threat and danger. It is the colour of dying plants.

Green is the colour of the abundant plant life upon which so much depends. In its perfect sense the colour is about life, renewal and growth.

However, in its opposite sense it is about envy.

And it is the colour of rot and decay.

Blue is the colour of the sky and the sea, and therefore it represents height and depth. In this way it represents expansion and space.

However, when the sky and sea seem to be close together and the colours blend so that there is no up nor down, then it can mean the limitation of dimensions as shallowness, restriction and constraint.

Indigo is the darkest colour in the rainbow. Dark blue is the colour of the peace at dusk. It shows the time for contentment, quiet and relaxation.

But it is a deep blue colour and it can describe the way people feel when they are sad. When somebody has 'the blues' it means that they feel the darkness and isolation of a long, dark night coming on.

Violet is the border between the seen and the unseen. Beyond violet colours cannot be perceived by people. So violet is about believing in something which is beyond our comprehension. It shows us the progression that happens into the unknown. Progress and belief is positive when it is for constructive purposes.

The contrary view is one of cynicism where we cannot accept anything beyond our own limited view. We can become closed to an acceptance of anything that is not made of stone.

And finally, the shape of the rainbow gives us an understanding of a bridge between two extremes. The connection between two opposite ends should be a beautiful thing rather than a confrontation. A bridge is for the connection of different ideas and people, rather than for their separation.

The rainbow is a sign to us that we should look for the brightness in all areas of life rather than the gloom. Perhaps that rainbow is the thing that can connect an old man to a young boy."

He looked at his grandson and smiled as he wiped away small tears from his, and his grandson's eyes.

21. THE WIND-BLASTED TREE

When the tree started to grow, it felt isolated. As it poked its growing tip into the air, it was disappointed. There it was, at the top of a wind-blasted hill where a bird must have dropped it as a seed.

It knew that it should be growing tall and straight, but the harder it tried to do so, the harder the wind seemed to blow.

Its roots had to dig deep into the soil and rocks to avoid the sapling from being ripped away by the gales. Its leaves had to hold on very tightly to the twigs and branches to avoid being torn off.

It felt that it was ugly because it was not perfectly shaped like the trees it could see in the river valley below. They were tall, balanced and lush. Birds used their branches to roost and nest. It seemed so very unfair that it was bent and crooked as it grew bigger. And this sense of failure made it stoop even more.

The tree wanted to be admired for its beauty, but it did not feel that beauty was ever attainable. It wanted to be appreciated for its height, but it knew that it would be stunted. Tall branches would be exposed and would be snapped off by the stronger winds.

It wanted to be useful for the birds by offering its branches to hold nests, but it was aware that building materials would be swept away before a nest could be finished.

But what it did not know was that animals, birds and the other plants admired this tree. They could see it from miles away and it became a landmark to help the birds to locate their nests and the land animals to get back to their lairs and dens. Even sailors used it as part of their compass to locate fishing grounds in the sea.

The tree was used in stories to explain the benefits of being tenacious despite adverse conditions.

It would always be explained to young ones in the same way. For example:

"If that tree can grow in such an exposed place, then think what you can do with a much better environment. See how it has adapted to cope with the wind, bending to go with the strength of the gusts rather than fighting back against a stronger force and suffering. Be like that tree. Use your ability to adjust to your surroundings in order to win."

Of course, the tree never heard such praise, and its parents were elsewhere, and unknown, so they could not encourage it to be proud.

One summer's day, the tree was aware of some people sitting in the shade of its branches, leaning their backs against its trunk. They were drawing and painting the view from the top of the hill, but not the tree. The tree felt that it was being used in order to allow the artists to capture the beauty of the landscape whilst at the same time turning their backs on the tree's ugliness. It felt sad. The artists were aware that there was a fine mist was in the air. They thought that it was the start of a sea haze, but it was a fine cloud of tears coming from the leaves.

The artists stopped their work and unwrapped some food. They walked around whilst eating and began to look closely at the tree. They discussed it, they admired it, they praised it so much. They talked about perseverance, determination and fortitude. They talked about it being a monument that was known for miles around. They said that the tree was the main reason for them climbing to the top of the hill.

Then, the tree felt so proud.

It was a strange thing, but from that day onwards, the people, birds, animals and the other plants all seemed to notice that the tree appeared to be standing taller and straighter.

22. THE VOLCANO'S STORY

The island rose gently above the transparent sea. Just beyond the white sandy beach, big trees stood like guardians. They looked, at the same time, outwards towards the ocean and inwards towards the island. The ground sloped up smoothly in the direction of a hill. It was the hill that seemed to be the very strength of the island. In the mornings, as its peak caught the first rays of sunshine, it became a beacon that signalled the new day to the world. As a place to live, it appeared to be perfect.

One day, a beautiful young girl, with long dark hair, looked across the sea from the island where she lived. She saw the other island. The Spirit of the hill seemed to speak to her, inviting her to travel to live together. After an argument with her parents on her island, she took her canoe and paddled to be in this new place. She arrived in the evening, just as the sun was setting. She pulled her canoe onto the beach, found a comfortable place to rest, and fell into a sleep. She had a wonderful dream about how the future would be in this new place; free from the squabbles on the island she had left. Then, early in the morning she heard a rumbling noise that she did not recognise, the island shook a little, but soon the noise settled down.

The next morning she found that her canoe had been damaged, so she knew that she would be stranded on the island, but it had been her choice to go there. She knew that she had to make the best of her situation.

Anyway, the days rolled by, most of them happy, some sad. She spoke to the hill but sometimes it appeared not to answer back, it seemed not to hear or to listen. Sometimes she enjoyed the company of the animals on the island, but sometimes she felt alone.

One day the hill started to rumble, quietly at first, but then the top blew off and rocks and lava spewed into the air, the peace and tranquillity were lost. Red-hot lava flowed down the hill for a day and a night, and then the volcano, as it now was, became quiet and remorseful, apologising profusely to the girl. The lava cooled down and the beautiful girl tried to carry on as before. She did not know why it had occurred, nor did the volcano. And, after this had happened a few more times, the girl became frightened. She never knew when it would take place again. She wanted to get away from the island but could not. So she planned and planned. She would build a new canoe to use if the volcano ever erupted again. Even when she was building it, the volcano appeared to know what she was doing and sometimes it still rumbled, but mostly, it was silent.

Time went by until she had built her canoe. Then one day she told the volcano what she was going to do, and why. The volcano was quiet, as if it were heartbroken.

The girl left for a new island where she thought that she would be safer. The volcano rumbled from the distance as if to remind her that her dream island was still there, although now stained by lava and fear. As if in anguish the volcano rumbled day after day, night after night. The girl heard the noise in the distance and knew that she had been right to get away. Even though the volcano was safe most of the time, her fear remained. The volcano became very lonely and sad. It had frightened away the most precious thing that had ever lived on its island.

In great sadness the volcano asked an owl that was flying overhead to find a healer to control the outbursts. The owl flew away and a few weeks later a wizard arrived on the island and proceeded to dig away at the top of the volcano. The wizard said it had to go away for a while and left the volcano to ooze without help, without any attempt to control the pain.

Lava flowed like tears and blood. The hurt and the pain that had been exposed went to the very centre of the Earth. This had all begun so many years before the girl had arrived. It started when the island was first born. The volcano was so full of shame and anguish that it wanted the whole island to sink into the sea, to be obliterated forever. Its only hope had been the girl who it had hurt so badly in the past. One night it erupted just to try to let the girl know how desperate it felt, but the noise and the smoke only frightened the girl. In the morning the whole world was covered in gloom from the black and acrid smoke, the echoes of the roaring were still in her ears.

So she covered her ears so that she could not hear the volcano any more; she covered her eyes so that she could not see the volcano any more. She hoped that it would go away forever. The volcano, so sad and so lonely, knew it had two choices. The first would be to live on its own for evermore. It knew that until the destruction caused by the explosions ceased, the island would never be safe again. The second option was to get help to stop itself from roaring ever again. It could cap the pent-up pressure from deep within. That should control the pressure that would destroy the volcano and the island if it the force were ever released again. The volcano knew that the girl had asked another wizard to cast a spell that if it roared again, it would sink into the ocean, never to surface again. The volcano knew at this point that it would never roar again in any event.

The volcano resolved to build and restore. It knew this would take time to do, but beauty was its only goal. The lava had cooled into rocks that would be used to rebuild the damaged landscape. New trees and bushes would grow, hope would take the place of anger, and love would take the place of fear. This would take time, so much time that, perhaps, the island could only be left as a monument to its dwellers of the future.

The night fell, and in the morning, the volcano woke up as the hill it had been in the beginning. The heat deep within, now coming from the warmth of its heart, turned its tears to a cloud that would crown it for ever more.

23. THE RIVER'S STORY

There once was a big river that had given life, sustenance and nurture to the lands that bordered it. It had done so for many years, but one day the Spirits of the river became angry because the land never seemed to thank the water for what it did.

The river cried so many tears about this that it overflowed, it burst its banks, and the plants drowned. The river was remorseful and the waters subsided. The plants grew back and everything returned to normal.

Then it happened again, and the river was apologetic once more. When the plants did grow back they were worried that it would happen again and again. And it did, but not as often. Still, it made the plants cast their seeds elsewhere to be safer, to be away from the unpredictable river.

Most of the time the flow was like the current of love, but when the river engulfed the land it was like an anger; uncontrolled and destructive. It intimidated the land.

Then one day the Spirits made boulders roll from the mountains. These stones blocked some of the tributaries and diverted the downpours from the thunderstorms. The river was now incapable of flooding, but most of the plants had moved away.

After a long time they learnt to hope again and the started to grow back nearer to the river, but they could never fully trust again.

24. STRAIGHT LINES

The old man sat by the river, thinking. He was pondering about the description his friend had given him.

"You're a very straight man" he had said. That meant he was honest. He wondered why an honest man was 'straight' and a dishonest one 'crooked'.

As he gazed across the gently undulating landscape he noticed that there were no straight lines in his field of view. The grasses he saw appeared to be upright but bent by the slightest of a breeze.

There seemed to be no straight lines in nature. In some ways, straight lines are fascinating, he thought. They are unique. They are human. All other lines are curved or bent. Of course, humans can make shapes like triangles, squares and complex multi-sided figures from straight lines. But, other lines make everything else.

He knew, after all, that everything is made from atoms. That is everything, not just us humans. He was talking to himself as if thinking out loud to his surroundings.

"Atoms are like little solar systems with minute charged particles orbiting each other. Those atoms make our cells and, the cells of every living thing. Those cells have a round, ball shaped, nucleus at its centre.

We exist on a planet that is ball shaped. That ball circles a round sun that, in turn, circles in a galaxy that spins in the Universe. Circles and curves are the shapes of our existence. Everything depends on circles and curves apart from the thinking of mankind which is becoming more and more rigid, and more and more a straight-line logical process.

There are few, if any, straight lines in nature. However, our buildings are based on straight lines. And our houses. And our offices.

Our learning is based on straight lines. Yes, only cause and effect counts. We spend our youth having to remember facts to pass examinations rather than for gaining knowledge or wisdom. Rather than learning about what life should be about.

We want to become 'logical and rational'. The flexibility and unpredictability of emotional and creative thought is reserved for the decorators of society such as the artists, writers and composers. But words are made from curving letters and music from waves of sound. Paintings rely on shapes and on perspective, the curvature of the Earth.

Those people who are supposed to have their feet flat, yes flat on the ground, look for the shortest route from A to B."

He snorted to himself.

"It is, of course, a straight line. But straight lines miss so much because they cover less ground. We just see less but we get directly to the point.

What is the point?" He thought.

"Curved lines are often safer, anyway. A zigzag path up a mountain side is far less steep than the direct route."

"So," he mused, "straight is about being rigid, whereas curves are about being flexible."

As he sat he wondered why his friend had insulted him so much by calling him a 'straight man', especially now, as when he was getting older he was becoming more and more crooked in his body.

He smiled to himself and then laughed to share his joke with the huge variation of shapes of nature around him, none of them straight.

25. THE WATER-WHEEL

The sun's energy turned the water of the sea and lakes into vapour which collected as clouds. This mighty weight of water looked light and fluffy as it floated in the sky, but a lot of energy had been stored.

When, sometime later, the clouds released the water onto the land, the corn growing in the fields, gave thanks for their drink. Not only did the rain provide refreshment, it also allowed the roots of the plants to absorb the dissolved minerals and other nutrients which were needed for growth.

The corn was not greedy, and the unused water ran away to make small streams that borrowed the energy of gravity as they flowed to the river.

The river collected a lot of energy as it flowed downstream. Other streams joined in, adding their vigour to the current.

When it got to a water mill, the wheel asked the river, very politely, if it would spare some of its energy to rotate it. The river was happy to give. After all, it had so much. And all of its energy had been given to it, anyway, so the river did not own its power.

The wheel was turned by the river, and it ensured that any water that was carried upwards, was returned to the flow. It was only the energy that was needed. The request was made every time the wheel turned, but the river never became bored because it changed constantly.

The water-wheel gave the force that it acquired to the mill-stone that turned to grind the corn. The stone was a little wasteful because it used some of the power to make heat and grumbling and grinding noises. However, it served it purpose quite well. And it owed its inefficiency to its design by humans who were very wasteful of natural resources, most of the time.

When the corn had been changed to flour, the energy of the water had been dissipated into different forms. The corn was just a carrier of the power that had been given by the sun, the rain and the earth.

The miller took that flour, added water, salt, sugar and yeast and used the sun's energy that had been stored in logs to bake it into bread.

That bread was sold, sliced and eaten to give vigour to its consumers. They in turn used some of that strength to tend to the land and its plants.

One day, some bread was left over and became stale. A man picked it up and took it to the river. Rather than waste all of the combined efforts that had been put into the loaf the man threw small pieces of it into the water to feed the ducks. One piece was missed and was collected by the current and taken downstream to the water-wheel.

That piece was part of everything that had contributed to its existence, as everything, in the Universe, that it knew was part of it. The connection was the flow of shared energy. Nothing in the whole cycle had been so greedy as to take what it had been given or loaned for its sole use. In this way the cycle could be repeated time and time again.

The river continued to flow onwards, taking water back to the sea to become clouds, rain and the catalyst for life. It was about to start its orbit all over again.

26. THE WAVE'S STORY

The water had eroded the base of the cliff over the years. The mass of rock fell; gathering speed as it descended. When it hit the ocean, a huge wave was born.

It travelled out to sea and began to settle down after the wrath of its violent birth. This particular wave was not sure what it was. It did not know how wide it was, or should be. It did not know how high it was, or should be. It was just a wave, just another wave surrounded by so many others, similar to itself.

It thought that it probably had a purpose, or else it would not have been created. It wondered what that purpose was. Much to its frustration, to a great extent, the progress of the wave was outside its own control. When the wind blew, it seemed to grow bigger and more powerful, even though it lost parts of itself as foam. Sometimes it became so big that the top rolled over and broke away. Even the hot sun seemed to steal parts of it to make clouds.

But when things settled down again, it was still the wave that it recognised as itself. It had changed but had remained the same. The wave had no way of dealing with this paradox.

The wave felt lonely from time to time. There were waves in front that never slowed down enough for it to catch up with, so that it could join up. Nor could it slow itself enough for the wave behind to merge.

Then there were times when it had fleeting contact with sea birds. It would lift them up with its front surface, and then lower them with its back. But this game only lasted for short bursts of time, while it rolled on past.

Now and again something would swim through it. A whale always disrupted it so much that it took a while to get itself back together again. The slash of a shark's fin, however, was easy to deal with.

The wave was perplexed one day when it realised that it was not a single individual piece of water moving, but something else. It was not like a fragment of seaweed that was being propelled across the surface of the ocean, but something that used the water to express its existence. It was an entity, but it did not understand how it related to the rest of the Universe.

It knew that it could be changed by the wind. The strong currents that lived in the sea could redirect it. It would grow whenever the seabed got close to it. It would even be pulled and tugged when the moon was at its brightest.

But what it was, it had no idea.

Then one day it came close to an island. It saw a strange creature that was neither fish nor bird. This creature was standing on what appeared to be a log. The wave was feeling mischievous and rushed towards the piece of wood. As it got there it concentrated on changing its pace by slowing and then rushing.

The man's canoe capsized and he was convinced that the foaming splashes were like the sound of giggling as the wave reformed itself and continued on its way.

The wave's feeling of pleasure was changing, however. It felt itself being lifted upwards. Its top was leaning too far forwards as its shape mutated into a curl. It was top heavy as it rushed towards the cliff. Big rocks on the seabed tripped it at its base, and it fell into the headland with a mighty crash. It knew that it was about to die and prayed that it would find peace in its afterlife.

Then, the wave was no more. Its body was smashed into little waves that were gobbled up by the maelstrom of heaving water.

The wave-of-sound from the collision of the breaker with the rock travelled out to sea and began to settle down after the wrath of its violent birth. This particular wave was not sure what it was. It did not know how wide it was, or should be. It did not know how high it was, or should be. It was just a wave, just another wave surrounded by so many others, similar to itself.

It thought that it probably had a purpose, or else it would not have been created. It wondered what that purpose was.

INSIGHT TO ANGER

27. THE ANGRY MAN

When the angry-man had first arrived in the foothills from his village, the thunder was shouting at the world. The language it used was unintelligible, but the tones suggested strength, power and danger.

Shortly afterwards, it was joined by the hissing of heavy rain. The water exploded from the sky to give sustenance to the few plants that it did not crush by its sheer force and weight. Yet, at the same time as being menacing, the storm was a comfort. The thunder was a noise that broke the silence and the lightning illuminated the area to give enough light to observe the damage from the deluge.

He never knew whether storms like this were a demonstration of anger, or if they were the forces of nature expressing their might in an arbitrary way. If it were anger, to whom did it belong? The black and solid clouds that were the parents of the thunder, the lightning and the rain moved slowly at the mercy of the wind. It was as if the gusts controlled where and when the storm would take place. It was as if it were the greater authority.

Yet sometimes the wind could be a soft and warm breeze like the breath of his wife's kiss upon his cheek in other times. Sometimes it could be a vicious and wild gale like the temper that he had let escape, and which had stopped those gentle kisses that he liked so much.

He wondered if the Spirits controlled the weather and the storms. If so, he tried to work out why they should be so angry. Was it the expression of the energy of the world? That intensity was so obvious everywhere. It could be seen in the rocks when they rolled down mountainsides to demolish whatever lay in their path. It was in the gushing of water in rivers, and waterfalls. It was in the flight of insects and birds.

It was in the movement of all animals. He found it difficult to think about where there was no energy. Even the dead gave their unused life to worms. And all this vigour came from the Earth, the Sun and the Moon. Everything was joined together in a huge web of energy. This must include him, and her.

The air always felt cleaner and fresher after the rains. There was always a purging as part of a tempest, but for him there was only guilt. So, he pondered, why did his relationship not get any better after his furious storm?

At this point, in desperation, he hoped that the lightning would find him to deliver its sudden and final punishment in an instant. A moment that he would be totally unaware of. But like all of his hopes, it seemed this one would also be left unsatisfied.

28. BLAME

The angry man wanted to resolve this conflict that lived within him. So he went to see the Wise Man who lived in the mountains. He told him of his childhood when he felt that his mother had been unkind to him. He thought that the anger he felt was the remains of the disregard that he had felt. He wondered if, when he became angry with the people he loved, he was really expressing the anger he would have displayed to his mother when he was a boy, but was too frightened to do so.

The Wise Man asked him if he thought the battle was between the man and his mother as she was now. Or between his younger self and his mother as she was when she was younger.

After a pause, he then asked if perhaps there had perhaps been a battle between her younger self and her mother who might have made her angry. And so he went on, back to the first mother on Earth. Then he asked the man if he would feel innocent or guilty if there were to be a battle between his children and himself as he had been.

He said: "Do their younger selves have a battle with you? And if so, whom should they blame? Themselves, their father, your mother, your grandmother, her mother, and so on? The only solution is to bring peace rather than retaliation. You thought you had found the reason for your anger in the way your mother appeared to be. But, remember that those are your thoughts and your memories, not hers. You saw the past through your eyes, not hers.

When memories are modified by our emotions they do not necessarily recall the truth. Anyway, why do you need to continue to blame others? That causes the conflict. It becomes a licence for bad behaviour.

If a single spark can burn a twig, and a single twig can burn a branch, and a single branch can burn a tree, and a single tree can burn a forest, and so on...what can you blame?

The only real action to take is to put out the fire before it destroys the world. Blame and hatred do nothing but destroy. Love and positive action are the only things that can extinguish a negative force. A firebreak, just one loving generation, will prevent the fire of anger from spreading. Blaming means nothing, but learning to control yourself is what brings peace, no matter what that takes. What you need to do is to destroy the anger rather than the person who might have caused it.

If you want resolution of your anger, then see your anger as an evil reptile. A symbol of the wrath within you. Destroy that rather than an image of your mother. Turn you negative emotions into something that you can deal with rather than allowing them to be amorphous things than can hide. It is up to you to extinguish the evilness within you, rather than the possible cause of it."

29. KILLING THE ANGER

The angry man felt himself being transported to a muddy swamp. He felt nauseous from the fetid smell of decay. His stomach heaved and he was sick onto the ground. The vomit was richly acidic, seeming to burn his nose. It was a pile of rotted, rather than digested, meat. It was sinking into the mud. After a while he became aware of a scaly rasping on his leg. It felt cold. Looking down he could see the tail of a large red and green lizard rubbing against him. It jumped around and its mouth was dribbling putrid saliva. Its eyes were red and yellow.

It seemed to be the very essence of nastiness. It was anger and jealousy in one being. And he felt disgusted that this creature had lived within him for so many years. He could feel the fear and the abhorrence that his wife must have felt whenever it surfaced. He felt so horrified that he wanted to return from his imagination immediately.

The man fought with the lizard as if he had the strength of five men. He kicked it, he hit it with a rock. He was not so much killing it as punishing it. He was seeking revenge on this thing, this symbol of his inner turmoil that spilled into his whole life. He was shouting, bellowing at the reptile. Then he rushed at the lizard, he picked it up and smashed it against the trunk of a tree. The lizard's back was broken, it was writhing in agony so much that it seemed that all of the misery that it had caused over the years was being re-lived in those few moments of its death throes.

When, at last, the creature collapsed onto the

ground, its death rattle filling the air, the man collapsed from his exhaustion and he just laid on the ground. His anger was dead, at last.

When he awoke, the Wise Man was standing close by looking at the corpse. The two men hugged. The man closed his eyes and sobbed uncontrollably. He felt different so he opened his eyes and saw his mother hugging him instead. Rather than recoiling he hugged her back. She was crying. She asked him if perhaps he will now forgive her for the way she was, in the same way that he hoped his wife would forgive him for how he had been.

The man stood back and told his mother that the thing he had learnt was that love was the most powerful force of all. It overcame hurt, anger and hatred.

What has happened in the past belonged to the past. The past was yesterday. We could only live in the present time and create our futures that way. They hugged again.

The twisted reptilian body was lying on the ground being consumed by ants and maggots. All of life recognised life and death. The lizard was gone as a living thing but in its death it was giving life back to the world, but life that was purified by the recycling that was the very essence of the movement of energy.

The monster had existed in him, not as a living thing, but as memories. It been kept alive by the energy of his own negative, jealous and destructive thinking. This demon had been created by thought, by reaction, by fermentation and by its freedom to express itself through his lack of control. In the end it had been destroyed by thought. Thoughts of love and hope.

30. POWER

The man asked the Wise Man how to obtain the power that he needed to change others. The Wise Man frowned. He said that to want power to change other people is about the manipulation of others for the benefit of the wielder of might. It is the same as bullying. He explained that the request goes against all of the principles that the man should have learnt about love.

He took the man to a place with four caves. He pointed to the one on the left. He said that the caves represented stages in time. He sat the man on the ground and started to explain.

"The cave on the left contains the past and you have spent so much time exploring that cave that, in essence, you are still living there. The second cave holds the present and the fourth one holds the future. Now, look into the cave of the past."

The man walked to the entrance of the first cave and looked in. He could see images flashing for fleeting moments. Then he felt different emotions rushing through him. They seemed like the mixture of misery and happiness that had been his whole life so far. That was certainly how his life felt at that moment. No future, no hope, no happiness.

The Wise Man told him that it was time to leave that cave forever.

They continued to the next cave. There, he could see and feel nothing but emptiness and desolation.

They walked to the fourth cave. It was also empty

The Wise Man spoke again. "The way to develop yourself is to dream of your future, and the way you dream it, is the way that it will be."

The man entered that vacant place and, in his mind, he pictured days of love and happiness. Days when the present time had been moved to the first cave, and the cave of the present was full of joy and peace. He could feel warmth, he could feel contentment. He could hear sweet words being exchanged. He left and thanked the Wise Man.

After a pause, the Wise Man asked the man to go into the cave that they walked past earlier. He said that it was the place of change, it was where the present and the future meet. He said that it was the source of the answer to the question that the man was trying to ask at the beginning.

He said; "there are two forms of power, not just one. There is the power which is for the control of others, and there is the power which is for the control of the self." The man nodded and then entered the third cave.

Suddenly it was as if a door had closed. The cave was pitch-black. The man could hear drums beating and the strange singing, almost chanting, of a word that he could not recognise, nor repeat. He sat on the ground. A voice spoke to him.

"Self control is about being able to let go rather than holding on. The one you love has strength because she walked away from you. You showed weakness by chasing her so desperately that you frightened her away. To gain strength you must learn to lose what you want in order to find what you need. What you want, at this moment, is a person who does not want you. What you need, for the future, is somebody who needs you.

The one you loved does not want you now, but in time she will need you when she has realised that you were more good than bad, and when she can see that your problems have been resolved. Then she will see that what you did for yourself, making those changes, were really for her. It came from your love of her.

You must accept that you do not need her, you only want her because you lost her. When you can walk away from that, and when she needs you, then the time will be right for you to ask if you still want and need her. If you do, then you can love each other again. If not, then you will have found your happiness anyway. If she will not understand why you were as you were, then you have lost nothing anyway!

In the meantime live your life for yourself, not for the person who does not want or need you. It is not your duty to be unhappy because somebody walks away from you. You have done everything that you can to remove those negatives from yourself. If that battle with your problems has brought about the results that you wanted, then celebrate.

However, if she ignores that conflict, if she does not want to see you as you have become, then it is better that you walk away because you are walking away from nothing. It only means that she has a war to fight within herself. You cannot fight that for her. Hold true to yourself and you will find the love that you deserve."

The voice faded. Light began to seep into the cave. The man felt confused and dazed. He left for the open air.

31. JUDGEMENT

The Wise Man led the man further into the mountains until they reached an entrance in the side of a hill.

The man entered a huge cavern. It was richly decorated with stalagmites and stalactites. They formed huge sculptures of breathtaking beauty. In the centre of this grand palace was a single triangular rock.

He felt overwhelmed with wonderment and fear. He was aware of the noise of movements towards this heart of life. Then a feeling of terror overtook him over and he scrambled onto the top of the rock. It seemed to him that this was the place of judgement, and as he thought of himself as guilty, he knew that he would be condemned.

A voice seemed to be coming from the stone. "There is no judgement here. There is no judgement in the Universe. When a lion kills an antelope there is nothing that will decide whether it was right or wrong, or whether it was killed cleanly or in pain. When a flower blooms there is nothing that decides whether or not it is beautiful. If a bear takes a man then the man's family would consider the bear to be evil and would want to kill it. The family of the bear, however, would think the man-killer to be good because he brought home food. Values of virtue can only exist in the minds of the judges, and that depends upon their point of view rather than a universal code of conduct or truth.

Mankind is unique in nature, however. It is the only living thing that believes that it has the right to judge. It is part of its character. So nothing is judging you apart from those people that you know; and yourself. The others have no power to change you, only to praise or rebuke. You, however, have the choice to make the changes that you need, and want to make, in order for you to be able to live in peace and fulfilment.

Your experiences have assisted you to deal with the wrath that lived within you and to see the way forward. They are unable to change the past, but they have enabled you to create a different future to the one which would have happened had you not chosen to alter your thought and behaviour."

"Who are you?" the man asked.

"I am your conscience. Use me, not to censure yourself, but to move forward from here.

You have to stop judging yourself so harshly. There are times when you can look at your behaviour and then change it to improve the lives of those you love if it is damaging. The only person who deserves judgement is the man who knows that he is doing wrong and does nothing to correct himself. This person has the problem because he does not care. You took the decision to change because you do care. It is so sad that the start of that process of transformation has caused so much heartache. Know that if those-that-you-took-that-choice-for cannot appreciate what you did, then perhaps they were not worthy of the torment that you went through for them. Perhaps they were, in fact, the fertilisers that helped the monster within you, to grow.

Sometimes, when you are a kind and caring person, who puts others' needs before your own, then you pay a high price. Those people that you have sacrificed everything for believe that their real place is in front of you. They lack understanding and appreciation. All they have learnt is how to be uncaring and selfish. Perhaps that is how those you loved had become. If so, then you do not need them and they certainly do not deserve you.

I have been here to help you to make the transition from the past to the future, to ensure that you have learnt from your experiences and your journeys. Let the future unfold as you wish it, and as it intends."

32. THE NEW DOMAIN

Suddenly, the man was floating through a tunnel in a shaft of pure light. He felt drawn by the attraction of exquisite sounds and visions. He was aware that his friends and relatives were preparing to greet him. He knew that he was travelling to a different reality where he would live in peace at last. He would be free from the torments of his life. He felt that, at last, he was becoming part of the Universe. He felt contented now. He knew that he would meet, love and be with his wife and his children again, but this time in a place where happiness, rather than hurt, would abide.

He floated into this New Domain, a place full of beauty and light. He saw something that was welcoming him. It was indescribable because it was not a person, it was not a Spirit, it was not the Universe, but it was something that was all of those things in one.

A beautiful voice spoke to him. "Welcome. You are not here for judgement because here, there is no judgement. You are here to fulfil what you want."

He pondered for a long time. He was attempting to bring his feelings together. There was joy at the thought that he was in a place where happiness was the norm rather than misery. At the same time he felt cheated that he had been unable to resolve his problems in his real world.

He replied. "I take it that this is the other dimension in which I shall now live. If it is, please listen to me. The Earth world was also a place of beauty, but that loveliness was not allowed to be expressed. There was hurt, there was pain and there was evil within the hearts of men.

Why, if you are the Great Universal Spirit, do you allow that to happen? If you live in all things then why do you not change the wrong-doing? Why do you need to torture us? It seems that the good people are punished for being good. Those who work, give and share, end up losing what they love the most. Those who are idle, those who take and hold are the ones who seem to have happy lives. It is not enough to say that there is no assessment here. There was assessment on Earth. Others judge the individual, and the individual judges himself. If the Spirit of the Universe lives in all things, then the Universe has an opinion of our worth. If we live in the Spirit of life, then surely we can be allowed to enjoy the Spirit of happiness and fulfilment before we come here."

He did not feel angry, but frustrated. His words felt more of a plea for man, animal and plant kind. He was answering the claim of being non-judgmental with an appraisal of the Great Spirit based on his own experiences. And if there were no judgements here, then he could not be punished for stating his point of view anyway! He continued.

"And now I will reply to what you said when I got here. So, this is a place where I can fulfil what I want! Well, I want to accomplish my duty as a good husband and a father, and a grandfather in time. I want to replace the misery that I gave my loved-ones with happiness. So grant me that."

The voice paused, and then answered. "Have you finished? I will assume so. What you had in your world was choice. That was freedom. You had the choice to carry the hurt from your life into the lives of others. Who do you want to blame for the options that you had? Do you want to be so controlled that you run your life as a stream does when contained by its banks, or would you prefer to have the freedom of an ocean?

What was really getting to you was that whereas you had the ability to decide how you would behave, you did not improve until you had to. And now that you have changed, you're upset because others have that freedom of choice about whether to take you back or to throw you away. You have learnt many things, but you have still not learnt to overcome your own disappointment in not being able to make people do as you desire.

I might be the fountainhead of all life, but I am not a wishing well. If I were then all beings could be as selfish as they want to be, as nasty as suited them, and then ask me for forgiveness. Everything would be without a conscience. As you said there are people who are knowingly selfish and who steal both emotional and material belongings from others. They have the choice to change as you did."

The man answered. "But what stops them from doing that? Are they ever punished if they are not judged?"

The voice replied. "Yes. They are punished by themselves because they never have what they want. If they have to take or hurt, then that is something that they feel they have to do. If they feel that they have to take something, then it is because they are suffering without it. Of course, once they have got something, then they will still need something else, and so on. In that way they are never happy. The people who are happy are the ones who give, freely and without conditions, something that they want to supply to make others happy. In that way happiness breeds happiness, misery breeds misery. And you have learnt that at first hand."

"So if I had been able to stop giving anger and the fear that caused, and had given pure love instead, we would all have been happy." The man stopped and waited in silence. "Is it too late now? Will I ever get the chance to give the love that I feel, but which has been obscured by the anger that has now been tamed?"

"There are two choices that you have now. You can stay here with your ancestors and the friends that you have lost, and feel the happiness that you seemed to have missed on Earth, or you can wake up in your life on Earth believing this to be yet another dream. You will have to be patient in order to live your dream, but one day you will return here anyway. Then we can talk again."

33. TIME

The man told the Wise Man about his

experiences. He asked the Wise Man to explain more about time because, if time did not exist somewhere, then there was the chance to erase, or change, the mistakes of his past. The Wise Man commenced his interpretation of his knowledge.

"Time does not exist as you think of it. The only time that there is, is the present. There is no future because the influences that create the future are in the here and now. If the present changes, then the future changes as well. The past is only a memory of how each point in time was. That cannot be changed because it has happened, and it therefore only exists in memories. Memories are just thoughts, and as thoughts change and mutate over time then actual events will appear to change as well. In this way the past that we know is only as real as a story that we have told. What do you remember from before you were born? Nothing more than you have been told, and that is not your experience, anyway. Stories are the thoughts of people that are changed and coloured to make them more entertaining, frightening or educational. We can never be sure that those stories are the truth.

Nobody can prove the truth, but the account that will be believed depends on the listener's opinion of the storyteller, not the facts.

For now, the thing to be aware of is that the future is changed by the way we are in the present. It is not changed by how we wish it to be, but only by believing how we want it to be in the future."

It almost seems too much for the man to understand. He could grasp that the way to change the future was to change the present, and the best way to do that was to change the one point of time that we are experiencing.

34. THE FOUR WORLDS

The man sat and watched as the Wise Man seemed to be working on the words that he would deliver. After a long he while started to explain.

"There are four elements; fire, the wind, the Earth and water.

There are four directions; the north, the east, the south and the west.

There are four forms of life; the animals, the plants, the elements of the rocks and Earth, and of course, the Spirits.

What you need to know now is that there are also four worlds. You saw those four locations of the Universe when you visited the four caves. You saw the past, the present and the future. The third cave is the one for advice and change.

What you were not told, but what you need to know was how to use that last cave properly. Follow me."

The Wise Man stood up and walked to the rear of the third cave. The man followed, his curiosity growing with every step.

At the very back of the cave there was a tiny hole in the ground. The Wise Man squeezed through and the man followed him. There were four tunnels leading in, and the centre stone was square shaped.

They stood at the first face that they saw as they entered.

"This is the here-and-now. Look carefully and you will see a reflection of yourself as you are; confused, questioning and lost."

They moved to the second face.

"This is the past. You can see the anger that you had. You can see its defeat. This face is about the retrieval of those things that were needed to be dealt with. Once those negatives had been retrieved then the reconciliation of those lost parts of your mind was achieved. The extinction of your anger took place and you were then able to be at peace with yourself and others."

The two men moved to the third face. The Wise Man said:

"This is where constructive advice is given to leave the past and to change the present to make a different future."

They then walked to the fourth face. The man could see the many choices that were available to him.

"One thing that you have been told many times is that you are responsible for your own destiny. Conceive your fate and it will happen. I will show you now."

The man looked closely at that fourth face and saw how in those earlier times, after he had quarrelled with his wife, he had started to think that his marriage was going to end. This belief widened the gap that started to grow. And after the next, and the next, and the next arguments, the gap became a valley, which then became a canyon.

"Can you see that what has happened is actually what you saw your destiny to be? And the actions that you took, allowing your anger to surface, just brought that destiny to reality?"

The man nodded his sad agreement. He looked glumly at the Wise Man and noticed that his friend was smiling.

"Why are you smiling at my downfall?" He asked, feeling very irritated.

"Because what you are watching is not only your downfall, but it is also your salvation. Can't you see? You now have the answer to your persistent question. How can you change somebody else for your own benefit? This was the revelation that you wanted. If you caused your current situation by your vision of this end, then you can change your life by assuming it to be the way you want it to be. If you really want to live your days out with somebody in harmony, happiness, security and love, then all you have to do is believe that outcome will happen, and no other. Your behaviour will change to fulfil your belief. That is why I am smiling. When you dream your dream, then your dream would come true.

We have all met people who have become ill because they think that they would succumb to sickness. There are also people who have lots of things because they think that they deserve them. The key thing to know is that we get what we think we will. We all control our own destinies; we shape our own lives. Who else would want to write scenarios for every living thing? Do you think that Spirits have nothing better to do? We are not handed a script at birth. Life is a play that we write ourselves.

We are all part of the Universe. What we want is what the Universe gives us. Regard the Universe as a container of all of the support that we need. The props for the play are available. All we have to do is to ask for those resources. Fate is the thing that seems to move you in the direction of fulfilling those dreams.

It seems strange, but when you are committed to achieving your future, then things appear to you. You find coincidences and omens. Helpful people seem to appear from nowhere. You find signposts. All you have to do is believe, not so much in an outcome that is preordained, but in your access, by right, to your share of the tools and assets of the Universe that will make your future come about. Know what you want to happen, and the resources that you need will appear. You are the one who creates that which will come to be.

"But isn't that using power for selfish benefit?" The man asked.

The Wise Man replied. "If we can live in these four realities simultaneously then we can live the lives that we choose rather than the ones that we fear we would live. You have great examples of this already. When you first met your wife, you dreamed that this girl would one day be your wife. When you married you knew that you would have children who you would be proud of. All of those positive things happened.

But when you doubted your marriage and your right to happiness, then you gave up your dream of restoring your marriage and it came to an end. You dreamed the end as it happened.

Then, when you applied yourself to resolving your problems, you knew that you would heal your anger, and so you did.

See and felt your dreams as new experiences rather than remembering your past. Only memories are from the past, you need to create a new future with new events.

Perhaps the Spirits have conspired to rid you of something else that you did not need, apart from your anger!"

The man nodded his acceptance of losing the past and of dreaming his future; to watch it come to pass.

35. RESOLUTION

When both The Wise Man, and the man, felt that he was ready, he left with a sadness in his heart, but a with spring in his step.

He said his 'thank-you's' and good-byes to the Wise Man and left the mountains. He returned by way of the foothills. There, the plants were growing in the sunlight. Saplings were appearing above the ground. Little animals scurried around.

Life had returned to this place, but it was new life that replaced the plants and creatures that had been destroyed. This place was about renewal. It was about the future springing from the past. The landscape would never be the same as it was before, but it would appear to new eyes as the way it had always been. The future was made from the present. The past was almost irrelevant.

The anger of the storm had destroyed what had been before, but it had allowed a new future to spring up.

At last, the man felt that he had purpose in his life. He was aware that much of his life to this point had been concerned with the destruction of things. His marriage, his family and his well-being.

He was thinking less and less about his wife and his sons. They had made no attempt to contact him and he started to understand that the problem that there had been had certainly not been one-sided.

The man dreamt his simple needs into being. When he wanted food or money, it would arrive as if by magic. Not in huge amounts, but always sufficient for his needs.

When he wanted company then people would arrive to chat with him. He had found the satisfaction that had escaped him before.

He continued to believe that one-day he would find the love of the person who would return his love. He hoped that his patience and care would be recognised by the Universe and communicated to this person.

He built his dream piece by piece with every day that passed, but felt frustrated that the one thing he really wanted seemed beyond his grasp.

He had learnt patience and consideration. He had discovered that trust comes from being honest, not only with the other party, but by being truthful to yourself. However, the man's dream was always the same. He wanted to share love and happiness with somebody.

Then, after the man was informed that his marriage to his wife had been formally annulled, he was upset, but not distraught. He knew that the water which crashes over a waterfall onto the hard rocks below becomes vapour that is taken back into the sky to become clouds, that become rain, that becomes water, that becomes the river at the top again.

And so his love, that had brought hatred of him, would be recycled to become love again. Not today, perhaps, but in the tomorrow of his hopes.

And time did go by. But he had grown weary of dreaming his dreams of a happy life with his ex-wife. Nothing had moved forward, there had still been no contact from her. He resolved to give up waiting for her, and to find contentment elsewhere.

After that decision, the man had a dream.

He felt that he was back in the mountains with the Wise Man.

Suddenly he could see the reptile he had killed so long ago. It was curled up like a dog in front of a fire. It woke up and smiled at the man.

The Wise Man told him to move towards it. The man felt scared. It was something that he did not want to see. It was, after all his anger. The Wise Man told him to sit down. Then, the reptile started to talk.

"I know that I worry you. We have had our differences in the past! Let me explain something to you about what I am.

Certainly I was created during your childhood as a result of the experiences that you had, and which were real. However, as you know, love is the thing that destroys anger. When you were married, the love you should have received was insufficient. That made you feel the same way as you did when you were a child.

That lack of love for you enabled me to grow. And as I got bigger so I was able to destroy the little bit of love that there was for you.

I am sorry, but that is my nature. I had to fulfil my role, if allowed to grow. It was not you that created and grew me, it was your childhood that planted the seed. Then it was your relationship that allowed that seed to germinate into what I became.

You destroyed me with the love that you held in your heart for other people, and now I am dormant in this comfortable place. What will happen is that you will now allow somebody else to love you as you should have been loved by your wife. As a result, I cannot grow inside you again!

There are many people who have an ogre of misery inside them, and those beasts can only survive by ensuring that they are in the company of others like themselves.

What seems to be a good idea at first, often develops into acrimony and sorrow. There is no way to deal with those monsters apart from by allowing love to smother them. But often, the bitterness that they cause makes the wounds too deep to heal."

The reptile then explained that, after a fire has raged and destroyed, the ashes may be used to bring nourishment to the soil

"Now that the fire of anger has burnt out, it will

help you to build rather than hurt." It finished.

The man woke with a start. His path was now easier to see, and to travel.

The man's new destiny became the one which, perhaps, he should have followed earlier, but had not, out of loyalty and duty to those he loved; those who still could not acknowledge what he had sacrificed for them.

A few months later, in his new village, the man said goodnight to the woman he loved.

At the same moment of time, his ex-wife wiped a tear from her eye and wondered what the man was doing these days. She was so lonely, so full of anguish.

She had dreamed her dream of being alone....and so she was.

Other publications by the author include:

BOOKS

The Secret Language of Hypnotherapy
ISBN: 978-0-9550736-2-5

Mind Changing Short Stories and Metaphors
ISBN: 978-0-9550736-4-9

AUDIO

Insight to Anger
Metaphorical stories about the destructive nature of anger and how anger can be overcome.

Stop Smoking
How to stop smoking easily and safely using hypnosis and breathing techniques.

Weight Control
How to reshape your body using hypnosis and visualisation. This method has helped thousands of people.

Fantasies and Dreams
Relaxation and positive thinking.

Self-Hypnosis
How to relax, visualise and set positive suggestions for yourself.

Animal Nature
Metaphors that relax and change the way you think based on animal stories.

Human Nature
Metaphors that relax and change the way you think based on stories about people.

Nature's Nature
Metaphors that relax and change the way you think based on stories from nature.

More information from: **http://www.emp3books.com**

Printed in the United Kingdom by
Lightning Source UK Ltd., Milton Keynes
140146UK00001BA/45/P